40 CATO ST

'A Fit Person t

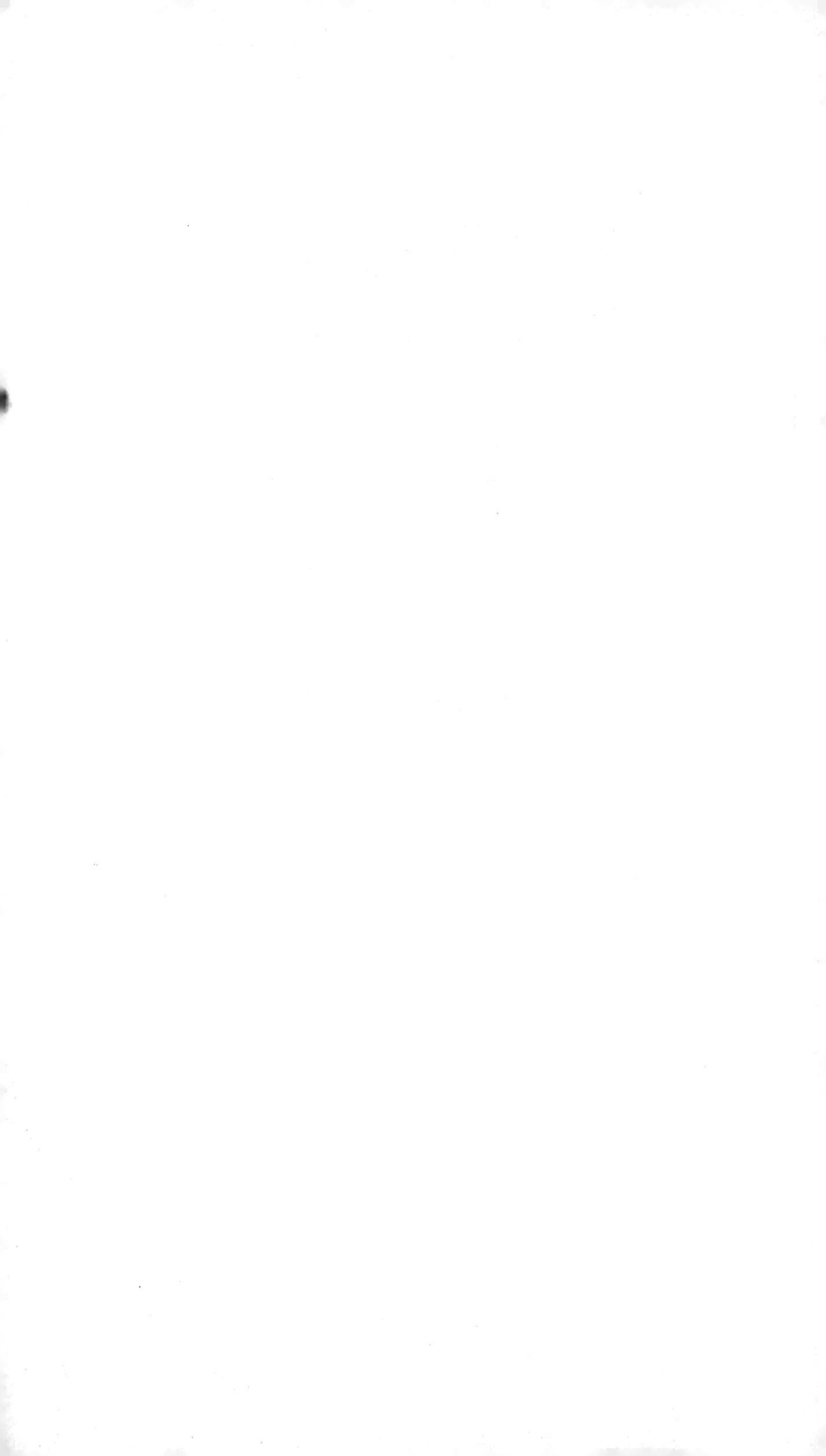

`A Fit Person to Be Removed´

Personal Accounts of Life in a Mental Deficiency Institution

Maggie Potts & Rebecca Fido

Northcote House

British Library Cataloguing in Publication Data

Potts, Maggie
 "A fit person to be removed": Personal accounts
 of life in a mental deficiency institution.
 I. Title II. Fido, Rebecca
 362.2

 ISBN 0-7463-0580-X

© 1991 W.J.M. Lovel (Nominee)
First published in 1991 by Northcote House Publishers Ltd, Plymbridge House,
Estover Road, Plymouth PL6 7PZ, United Kingdom.
Tel: Plymouth (0752) 705251. Fax: (0752) 777603. Telex: 45635.

All rights reserved. No part of this work may be reproduced or stored in an information retrieval system (other than short extracts for the purposes of review) without the express permission of the Publishers given in writing.

Typeset by Concept, Crayford.

Printed and bound in Great Britain by Billing & Sons Ltd, Worcester.

Contents

	List of Illustrations	vi
	Acknowledgements	vii
	Introduction	9
1	'A fit person to be removed' *Admission to the colony*	13
2	'Colonies: homely and simple' *The ideal system*	24
3	'What have I come to?' *First impressions*	36
4	'They treat us like children!' *Routines, rules and regulations*	45
5	'You did anything wrong — God help you!.' *Ensuring obedience and respect*	57
6	'I've worked all me life up till now' *Creating useful colonists*	67
7	'On certain days, certain times, certain nights...' *Leisure and special events*	80
8	'There was some just hiding their feelings' *Social and sexual relationships*	100
9	'Half me life's been wasted' *Changes and freedoms*	115
10	'It's all changed'	130
	Appendix I: The Mental Deficiency Act 1913	140
	Appendix II: Brief biographical details	146
	Index	151

Illustrations

Cover	The 1943 laundry which washed, pressed and folded more than 10,000 articles each week.	
2.1	'There will be no justification for the expenditure of large sums of money.' Dormitory accommodation, circa 1940.	28
2.2	'There were wooden chairs and pipes and a big old-fashioned fireplace.' Day room on a villa for sixty 'high grade' female patients.	28
6.1	The first schoolroom, 1922 for: 'Those patients who are able to benefit by the simpler forms of kindergarten occupations.'	69
6.2	The colony school, 1947: 'Improving those damaged and shapeless lives.'	69
6.3	The stone sinks for hand-washing clothes and towels, which provided employment for less able female patients, 1943.	73
6.4	Preparing the ground for spring, circa 1935. Note new boundary wall.	73
7.1	A villa for the 'lowest grades' to accommodate twenty males and twenty females. Official opening, 1932.	85
7.2	'The Recreation Hall provides seating for six-hundred persons and is intended to form the centre of the social life of the colony.' Official opening, 1941.	85
7.3	Scout gymnastic display at the colony sports day, 1948.	93
7.4	Colony Christmas cakes, circa 1950.	93

Acknowledgements

We are especially grateful to **Lorraine Day**, not only for her skills as an interviewer, but also for arranging and organising readings of the book. We could not have managed without her enthusiasm and commitment which have been essential to the successful completion of the project.

Thanks are also due to **Steven Ward**, **Gaynor Hollis** and many other staff for the time and care they have taken in recording memories of life in the institution. Also our thanks to **Kay Mellor** for reading aloud each chapter to the men and women who took part.

This project could not have been undertaken without the financial support of the Health Authority nor its willingness to expose to public scrutiny the history of one of the services for which it is responsible.

Finally, we owe our gratitude most of all to the men and women who took part in this project and who have taught us so much. This book is about them and their lives and is dedicated to them and to all people who continue to be the victims of our care systems.

Introduction

The major reorganisation of the social and industrial life of Great Britain in the late eighteenth and nineteenth centuries produced its quota of victims. The Industrial Revolution resulted in increased complexity of work in factory, foundry and mill. Those who found themselves unable to work in these changed circumstances, people who were old, young, disabled, mentally ill or handicapped, became public responsibilities; they were cared for in public institutions, the most common and the most feared being the workhouse.

The first attempts to provide for the specific needs of people with a mental handicap in the early part of the nineteenth century were largely humane and far-sighted, being rooted in the belief that such people required and would benefit from structured education. The enthusiasm and optimism of some of these early pioneers was reflected in the development of schools and colonies which embodied a positive humanitarian approach to individual development and training: mentally handicapped people were considered to be human beings like the rest of us. 'An idiot is endowed with a moral nature and is influenced by the same things as the rest of humanity' (Seguin, 1846)[1]. Unfortunately, this early humanitarianism and optimism did not survive the social changes begun by the Industrial Revolution and it is not until a hundred years later that Seguin's words have been echoed by the modern pioneers of de-institutionalisation and care in the community. 'Mentally handicapped people have the same human value as everyone else' (Kings Fund 1980)[2].

The dividing line between normality and mental handicap is socially and culturally determined. In the intervening hundred years, the harsh effects of social change, the break-up of families and social networks and the ethos of work or starve, resulted in many people who could not be cared for within their family. From the mid-1850s until relatively recently, services for people with a mental handicap have been dominated by the belief that mental handicap is a major social evil requiring containment and control. Medical interest at the turn of the century into the causes of crime, immorality and poverty laid the blame on mental handicap. The early work of psychologists on the nature of intelligence resulted in an emphasis on its inherited and unchangeable

---

[1] Seguin, E. *Traitement moral, hygiène, et éducation des idiots et des autres enfants arrières* Baillière Tindall, 1846.
[2] *An Ordinary Life: Comprehensive Locally Based Services for Mentally Handicapped*

nature. People with mental handicaps therefore became the convenient scapegoats for the ills of society. The solution was simple: exclusion and prevention became of paramount importance. Confinement and rigid segregation of the sexes were the guiding principles.

Mary Dendy[3], an active campaigner writing in the 1890s, believed that children classified as mentally handicapped should be 'detained for the whole of their lives' as the only way to 'stem the great evil of feeble-mindedness in our country'.

Views such as these fuelled the demand for new public institutions with such effect that the number of asylums created for idiots increased from four hundred in the mid-nineteenth century to almost two thousand by 1914.

Prejudice was rife: 'Feeble-minded women are almost invariably immoral and if at large usually become carriers of venereal disease or give birth to children twice as defective as themselves. A feeble-minded woman who marries is twice as prolific as the normal woman...Every feeble-minded person, especially the high-grade imbecile, is a potential criminal needing only the proper environment and opportunity for the development and expression of his criminal tendencies. The unrecognised imbecile is the most dangerous element in society.' (Fenald, 1912)[4]

It is within this pessimistic context that the Mental Deficiency Act 1913 came into force. It reflected society's view that it should be protected from the evils of mental deficiency. The Act permitted the certification and detention of people on the ground of their level of handicap, defined as idiocy (severe), imbecility (moderate), feeble-mindedness (mild) or on the grounds of moral defectiveness.

Although there was much debate in Parliament about the proposed Act and its effect on the liberty of the subject in the writings of the time, people who were classified as mentally handicapped were considered to require care and protection rather than liberty. The liberty from which they required most protection was, in the view of society, the liberty to 'repeat their type' and thus increase the numbers of the 'degenerate and wastrel classes, with disastrous consequences for the entire community' (Wormald and Wormald, 1913)[5]. The Act provided for the paternal protection by the state of those who were in effect viewed as perpetual, and sometimes wilful, children.

---

[3]Dendy, M. *Feeble-mindedness in Children of School Age* Manchester University Publication No 13, 2nd edition, 1920.

[4]Quoted in Sarason, S.B. and Doris, J. *Psychological Problems in Mental Deficiency* 4th edition New York, Harper and Row, 1969.

[5]Wormald, J and Wormald, S. *A Guide to the Mental Deficiency Act, 1913* King and Son, 1914.

It was against this background that the colony referred to in this book as 'The Park' was conceived and designed. Having been delayed by the advent of the First World War, it was officially opened on Tuesday 3 June 1920 at 3.00 pm by the Chairman of the Board of Control in the presence of the Lord Mayor and other members of the County Council. The colony fulfilled an 'insistent local need' to provide institutional care for the 'most helpless members of the community'. According to the programme for the official opening, the institution had been 'especially organised for the reception of the imbecile and idiot class of defectives who in many cases suffer from epilepsy and physical infirmity' and who were certified under the Mental Deficiency Act 1913.

The Park was considered an ideal system: it was planned to consist of small houses or pavilions around a central block, thus enabling different classes of inmates to be cared for separately and representing a considerable improvement on the large single building type of institution. The Park 'stands on high ground in a retired and healthy position and is a composite picture of parkland and woodland with charming rhododendron walks and well-stocked gardens of vegetables and fruit trees.' The design of the colony at that time was no doubt based on the views of the two most influential local officials:

> There will be no justification for the expenditure of large sums of money in erecting costly and palatial buildings as in the case of many Asylums or other similar Public Institutions in the country. Colonies, homely and simple in character and free from unnecessary repressive and restraining methods, with a large acreage of land and timber, and where the patients can be employed under competent overseers in the various branches of agriculture, should be provided.[6]

This then was the background to the opening of The Park. The purpose of this book is to continue its history through the eyes of the people committed to spending their lives within its boundaries. How did they perceive the charming position of The Park, its routines and its treatment of them? Some of the residents admitted under the 1913 Act are articulate and anxious to talk about their experiences of life in the institution. The idea of recording these experiences arose from conversations in an advocacy group and in a club for elderly residents. Current concepts of community care envisage the closure of the large segregated institutions but the memories of those who were certified under the 1913 Act and who experienced life in these institutions at first hand should not pass unrecorded. These memories are a valuable source

[6]Wormald, J and Wormald, S., op. cit.

of historical information which may prevent society from repeating the mistakes of previous care systems.

The eight men and nine women who took part in this project were anxious to tell us about their life in the colony. Except for one person, all were admitted under the 1913 Act. Most were admitted as children or as young adults, the average age being seventeen. The youngest was admitted one month before her fifth birthday. Between them, these seventeen people have spent an average of 47 years in the institution: the length of stay varied between 25 and 63 years.

During the three years this project has taken, we have met together regularly to read aloud each chapter as it was written. Every reading has stimulated yet more memories and information. As people have talked, they have learned to value their own history and become increasingly confident and determined that the public should know what life has been like for them.

For the authors, the writing of this book has been an enlightening and, at times, uncomfortable experience. It has forced us to recognise the humanity and uniqueness of people labelled mentally handicapped and has left us struggling to reconcile this to the fact that we are employees of a system which still, to some extent, wishes to deny such knowledge.

1

'A Fit Person to Be Removed'
Admission to the Colony

When I left school I worked at Freeman's. It's going back since I was seventeen. I worked up until I got intro trouble. I didn't go home 'cos they knew I was in trouble — they knew what had come. When I did go home, she (mother) said, 'If you are having a child,' she says, 'I won't have neither the child nor you near me doorstep!'

I was out all night and then I went home. Door was locked so I went down 'cellar. And in those days with coal, you know coal fires, I slipped down 'wall grate and got in that way. And just as I got to 'top o' steps me brother and uncle were on 'step wi' belt. Gave me such a good hiding cross 'back, sent me out again and locked 'door again.

And then I were out all night. Executive Officer went to Freeman's to see if they'd have me till it were born. Then when it were me last day, he came and said I were going home. Instead of taking me home, he took me to another hospital and I never saw me mother and father.

In March 1927, a couple of weeks after Elizabeth's eighteenth birthday, she gave birth to a baby girl.

Well, me elder sister went down and took her from me when I were in hospital. I didn't know me sister was going to come for it. I thought I was going to get it all over, meself better and when it were time to go home I was going to take her with me. I didn't know nothing — anything about it. She brought her up as hers, had her name changed and everything. To think I've never had her, with her bringing her up, 'cos that hurt me more than anything. Well I cried and cried — I couldn't help it. And there's been hours I've been in bed at The Park on villa 4, cried me eyes out.

Following these events, Elizabeth was certified as 'feeble minded'. In assessment, she was reported as 'Although eighteen years of age, she is childish in behaviour, breaks into a fit of weeping when questioned, will not look up and is persuaded only with the utmost difficulty to answer questions.' Elizabeth was judged to be emotional and unstable, easily moved to tears or smiles and unfit to hold her own in the world. On the same day, a petition for an order to send her to an institution on the grounds of neglect was signed by the Executive Officer. The

Statutory Declaration and Statement of Particulars to accompany the petition was signed by the Executive Officer and Elizabeth's father five days later. The next day, four months after the birth of her daughter, the order to send her to an institution was signed by a magistrate. Two days later, she was admitted to the local Institution for Girls. After five years, she was transferred to The Park Colony and has remained there since, spending more than sixty years of her life in institutions.

Horace went to an ordinary school before being sent to special school. He only stayed in special school for five months. When he left there he went to an Occupation Centre for Ineducable Children. From there he went to a tailoring department at an Industry Centre.

> I used to work at a tailoring place. You know, these waistcoats, putting lining inside, well I had to put canvas into a waistcoat. That's when I was sixteen. We only use to get 1s. 6d. a week and that weren't much to me.
> Me mother couldn't cope with me 'cos you see, she got rid of one of the beds that I was sleeping in and that's why I went into The Park Hospital.

Horace was classified as an imbecile when he was seventeen years old. Assessment of his ability stated that he could read haltingly and unintelligently and could only manage the shortest and easiest words. Assessment of ability seems to have been crude and rather arbitrary. For example, Horace was asked to differentiate between a fly and a butterfly and also between a stone and an egg. His response to these questions was described as 'inadequate'. Horace was condemned as naïve and childish'. The fact that 'when taken away, he cried like a child' only served to confirm the diagnosis. Three weeks later, three days after Christmas, he was admitted to The Park and remained there for thirty-two years.

Ernest, having been born with a congenital handicap, spent most of his childhood in various hospitals.

> I was in there because of my condition, my childhood illness.

When he was sixteen years of age, the general hospital felt they were unable to help him further. He was judged to be undeveloped intellectually and was officially certified one year later and placed on the waiting list for The Park.

> Well it was the General Hospital where I was visited. The person who came to see me a week before I came in, he told me that it was a change from the other hospital that I had been in since my childhood.

In assessing Ernest, no account seems to have been taken of his long period of hospitalisation. For example, his defect was related to his lack of knowledge of current affairs, of money values, of weights and measures and of arithmetic (e.g. 8 + 7 = 13). However, Ernest himself says:

> I read for the first time when I was only five years old. As far as my writing is concerned, I learnt that in two ways; in writing letters in print, I was taught that by my cousin. As far as real writing is concerned, I learnt that from a fellow patient in The Park and partly from letters I used to receive from my late father.

Ernest does not appear to have received any formal education: he has taught himself many basic educational skills. He learnt to read prior to his admission to The Park and has continued to develop and expand these skills. He wrote an account of his life in hospital which is now in the hospital library. One member of staff observing Ernest's progress some years later writes: 'He is an excellent reader with a good understanding of what he has read... If indeed he is self-taught, he has achieved quite a remarkable standard'.

Margaret spent the first few years of her life in a children's convalescent hospital. She suffers from cerebral palsy and cannot walk. At the age of four she was judged unable to benefit from education.

> I came in here because I couldn't walk. I were only a baby then. I couldn't talk or anything.

She was assessed on two occasions, the first time when she was nearly four and the second when she was almost five years old. Despite her physical handicaps, Margaret did make progress during this year, learning to sit up and to say more words. However, this was insufficient to prevent her being deemed incapable of receiving education at school and she was transferred from convalescent home to colony at the age of five years. Margaret's possessions which were sent from the convalescent home a few days later were listed as:

1 coat
1 dress
1 cardigan
1 pair knickers
1 vest
1 pair socks
1 pair shoes

Joan too was physically handicapped: at the age of eight years she, like Margaret, was stated to be ineducable because she was unable to walk and had a speech defect. Her physical handicap resulted in Joan having constant involuntary movements and spasms: during assessment, however, she was described as 'restless and inattentive'. This official also recorded that, 'When I asked her how many noses she has, she simply giggles foolishly, grimaces and wriggles about in her chair.' Because of her physical handicaps, very little assessment of her abilities seems to have been made, the definition of defect resting almost entirely on her physical limitations. Up to the age of eight, Joan had lived at home.

Me mam and dad were getting on... they were very happy with me.

Her speech is still difficult to understand but her friend Margaret understands it and interprets for her.

Sometimes people can't understand what she says and I help her.

Joan was judged as needing supervision and training of a type not available in her own home or in a special school. She was therefore admitted to The Park where she has since lived for more than forty-five years.

George suffers from a medical condition which results in constant, uncoordinated muscular movements that involve his entire body. This condition makes it very difficult for him to exercise control over his limbs, his tongue, his lips and his head movements. Not surprisingly, therefore, he failed at the age of eight to pass the Medical Officer's assessment. He could not stand alone nor wash, dress or feed himself. His determined efforts to communicate with people who talked to him were dismissed as 'dribbling with excitement when spoken to'. There is not one positive statement in the entire assessment and no acknowledgement of the inevitable effects of such a handicapping physical condition on his development.

George was classed by one official as an idiot and by another, who assessed him on the same day, as an imbecile. George was only eight years old at the time but the date of his admission is etched in his memory as some twenty-four years later he was able to recall it correctly when asked. The statement summarising the main findings concluded that George had no speech, was doubly incontinent, needed all nursing care and 'will need to be in hospital for the rest of his life'. He did in fact remain in hospital for thirty-six years before achieving that goal towards which he had worked with single-minded determination, his discharge back into the community. He now lives in a ground-floor flat which he shares with his friend Tom.

Sally worked in a mill from leaving school until she was nineteen years old.

> When I worked in 'mill and I were only getting 35 shilling and I said t' overlooker, 'Can I have some more money?' and he said, 'No, you can't.' He said, 'You can take your cards and clear out!'

She was admitted to The Park towards the end of the war. 'The Park' seems to have been used as a kind of bogeyman in her parents' attempts to restrict her.

> I was brought there 'cos I wouldn't get up for 'mill. And me mother put me there 'cos I wouldn't do as I were told. Me mother weren't too keen on me, but me father were different altogether. He used to spoil me and me mother were 'opposite.
>
> Well, how it started because she saw me at 'pictures with a boy and she came spying on me and she saw me and said if you don't come back home wi' me you're off to The Park. So she did it, she got me here. That's the place where they punish you if you're naughty!
>
> If she hadn't got me to The Park, we might've been married. I never saw him again. I think that were awful! I were just getting on nice and then me mother put me there. That were 'first time I'd seen him at the pictures and he said, 'We'll go for some fish and chips when we go.' And I didn't get them!
>
> I knew what were going to happen when she said, 'If you don't come home you're going to The Park'. So I said, 'Well, I'll go home.' But she still got me there.

Administratively, the reasons for an individual coming into the institution related to one or more of the following: lack of ability, inability to work, or family social and financial circumstances, which were sometimes detailed extensively, incomes and outgoings being taken into account. All who took part in the interviews had a good understanding of the immediate reasons why they came into the colony. Many of them also had vivid memories of life before their admission.

> Me own home were in A. . . Me father gave it up and I went to live with me aunt. Well, all three of us, two aunties and me father altogether. They were school teachers. One went to school and the other was a home marker looking after me and me father. He was still working then.
>
> When me mother died there were nobody to go to. I could've gone to Birmingham but it were too far for me father to go. He wanted to come and see me. Others were too far away than that; Stoke, Birmingham, Southport.

They brought me to The Park because it were the nearest one to come. (Doris)

Me mother and me went to (the workhouse) and they moved me mother. She died, so I went into The Park. (Elsie)

My mother died and there was no-one to care for (me). . . I had to stay — I had no mother. (Enid)

I were at home with me mother and sister and brother. I must have been fifteen or summ'at like that when (I came in). I left social services when I were fourteen years old. . . to work in t'mill. I did spinning and weaving. I only got ten shillings a week but to me it were worth it. I've no idea at all (why I come into The Park). I can never find out. Anyhow I'm not bothered. It could be, as they say, I were black sheep o' family. They've all died now that's why I can't get to know nothing. (Grace)

I lived at home. That's when my parents were living then, you see. I went to the Lane School. I went morning and afternoon and headteacher gave me a good hiding. I couldn't tell you why or anything. So when it was time to go home, I went home and told me mother about it. Next morning me mother went up worrying, to see 'headteacher. So my mother wouldn't let me go there any more so I went to another school. I was there until I was old enough to leave it.

I went (to work) with one of my sisters, where they used to pack lucky bags with sweets and that in. They were ha'penny ones.

When they (parents) both died I had to come here. I wasn't capable to look after myself. The doctor told our Mary. Our Mary asked if I were capable to look after myself but 'doctor wouldn't hear of it. Doctor told our Mary, 'No she isn't quite capable to look after herself.' I couldn't tell you why or anything. (Violet)

I used to go to special school and they (parents) were packing sandwiches for me. . . to take for me dinner and then come home and have a hot dinner. (David)

We were very poor. Nice and clean and we were well looked after. Them days you'd no money that's why. They hadn't the money to make a fancy home. (Grace)

Only George makes any direct reference to mental handicap.

I was backward.

The notes made as part of the certification procedure contrast sharply with the memories recounted. Perusal of the old records recreates starkly the spirit of the Mental Deficiency Act 1913. In assessing defectiveness, no account is taken of age, personal circumstances, individual experiences or reactions to the trauma of being 'examined'. Judgements were based only upon facts elicited at the examination and with no apparent concern even for those of tender years about the effect of what must have been an alien and unnerving experience. The terms 'childish' and 'cries easily' are used frequently. Behaviours such as restlessness and inquisitiveness noted at examination of young children (seven years or younger) were simply viewed as evidence of mental defect. Smiling is viewed as inane or unintelligent (even in a four-year-old): nervousness or lack of confidence or simply the desire to appease or to please are not considered as possible causes.

The criteria employed for assessing 'feeble-mindedness' appear to change arbitrarily to justify the label. For example, answers to questions such as 'Where is France?' — 'Over the sea'; or: 'Name some towns' — 'Bradford and Batley' are viewed as inadequate and provide only a further demonstration of mental defect. The scorn with which these answers are treated is apparent even in the official documents. Many of the questions posed in that formal atmosphere must have struck the candidates as distinctly odd.

> She is unable to see any absurdity in several statements containing obvious ones.

In making the diagnosis of mental defect, official evidence is essentially a list of wrong answers to questions of general knowledge.

> He fails to form a sentence with three given words. He fails to multiply by seven, to state the number of half-crowns in 15s. And to correct a slow clock. He fails to state similarities in an apple and an orange, to repeat five digits backwards and to solve a simple test of reasoning.

For many people brought before the examining doctors, this failure to give enough correct answers ensured certification as 'a fit person to be removed' to an institution.

No account is taken of the effects of prolonged hospital care, bereavement, poverty or physical handicap on child development. Inability is vested within the individual. The child was judged at examination and the label 'imbecile' or 'feeble-minded' applied. The prime aim seems to have been to justify formally admission to the colony. Opinions are pessimistic and the majority of statements made about people concentrate on what they are unable to do. Even where more positive comments are made, they are phrased in ways which emphasise defect: 'He is a harmless, droll, pleasant little fellow.' Those comments which refer to character and personality are largely emotive and damning: 'wayward', 'untruthful', 'dishonest'. One young woman was described as 'untruthful, dishonest, of doubtful modesty, clean in appearances'. Evidence for these terms is lacking and such statements stand as an all-embracing description of the individual. Society in the earlier part of the twentieth century was content to judge, label and dispose of people.

Under the Mental Deficiency Act 1913, local authorities had two main duties to fulfil. They were to see that certification of all people considered mentally defective took place and to set up special institutions for those who were thought not to be receiving adequate care and/or supervision at home. Local authorities established Mental Deficiency Act Committees to ensure that these obligations were carried out. A National Board of Control monitored the progress and work of these Local Committees. The Local Committees employed a specially approved part-time doctor to carry out examinations for certification. They also employed an Executive Officer who was responsible for 'ascertaining' potentially certifiable adults and children. Many can remember this man well as he was the one who visited the family, arranged the medical examinations, and saw to all the paperwork and the judicial orders before taking the person himself to the certified institution. Because of his role, most statements made about Mr Grey, the Executive Officer, reflect the anger, anxiety and unhappiness that the certification procedure and subsequent admission caused.

> Mr Grey, he took me up in his car from home. I called him a sneaker. He took me to 'hall. Mr Grey wanted my father to pay for me up at The Park. My father told him where to get off. He put me there, I've been there ever since.

> It was a man what sent me. A man called Mr Grey. He was bringing lads in.

> Mr Grey (took me). He was my welfare supervisor, you know, a person who owns the place, what goes visiting round.

> A man took me to The Park. It wasn't me mother. Me mother was looking for me.

The following account reflects the feelings of being marked down and trapped by the system.

> Grey! Oh blow that bloomin' thing! I used to go running to me mother. Mind

you, they used to come down that street and make you come out of the door. Ooh I hated him! He weren't only after me. He were clever. He got hold of nice girls in there. They were just like me.

You wanted someone with you, not just your mother, someone higher up to stick up for you. He (Mr Grey) put damper on me and told lies about me.

You weren't allowed to talk to Board of Control unless they talked to you.

What could you do! Family had to go with you. I felt awful. I worked at a mill, they complained that a man picked me up.

It is no wonder that the Executive Officer was referred to by one and all as the 'rat-catcher'. Frank remembers this well:

Got fetched here by that rat-catching fellow. 'Cos he were always picking young kiddies up and fetching them up to The Park. I weren't scared of him. Me uncle took me there and told me I were going somewhere, I didn't know where and it were blinkin' office to see Mr Grey.

'What's been happening?' he says.

'There's nowt happened', I says, 'It's them, they are trying to put me away.'

Well he let me go but I don't know what he said to them, but he let me go back home. It were a bit after when he come. He got me and he took me to The Park. I were here before my time, I were!

I were right mad about 'em! Me aunty, she fetched me in, she did a lot of it.

I felt upset, I couldn't stick it here!

as does Grace:

There were a certain man, used to pick people up. He's dead now — thank goodness! He wouldn't let anybody live. He did a lot of damage, picking up people what didn't deserve to be picked up. Every time they saw him, they called him that — 'the rat-catcher'. I used to hate him!

The officer's handbook[1], a practical guide to the Mental Deficiency Act, gave the following advice to Executive Officers when conducting the certification procedure in front of a magistrate.

Again it is stressed that the proceedings should be informal and every effort made to produce a homely and humane atmosphere throughout the hearing. A straightforward petition with the parent's consent only takes a few minutes, but 'awkward' cases need unhurried consideration. A conscientious judicial authority will appreciate this and take care to carefully read the medical certificates and depositions. One should avoid if possible the Justice, and

---

[1] Hoyle and Hawksworth, T.S. *An Authorised Officer's Guide to the Administration of the Lunacy, Mental Treatment and Mental Deficiency Acts and Regulations* Elsworth Brothers Ltd., 1948

there are some with little interest, whose attitude is briefly 'Yes, where do I sign?' and which creates in the parent's mind a very haphazard way of dealing with what is to him a most important problem.

All officers must establish a friendly and sympathetic bond between themselves and the patients they care for.

The Mental Deficiency Act 1913 made provision for the order for institutional care or guardianship to be renewed or revoked at the end of the first and second years and subsequently at five-yearly intervals. This procedure also involved appearing before a formal committee.

> When doctor were here he used to have a committee for our people to come up and see if they could get out. Committee doesn't come up now like they used to do when doctor was here.

It is difficult to imagine the certification procedure or its renewal being a relaxed and informal occasion, either for parents or for potential inmates. This must have been especially so since one of the major motivating factors for colonising people who were considered mentally defective was to ensure care and control at minimal cost. This required that a proportion of the inmates were able-bodied and capable of carrying out the day-to-day work of the institution. It is quite possible that, consciously or unconsciously, there was a reluctance on the part of such formal committees to allow useful workers to leave the institution.

> It is not true what was written down. They just did it to keep us locked up so that people would think we're mental.

> I used to go to the Town Hall. You know for the Magistrate. They used to say questions but *he* were always there butting in. They'd have let us out free but he were always there. Parents that come with us could never get their say — 'cos he was always butting in. Same with the Committee at The Park. Used to have a Committee every so often when parents used to come up to the Hall. Well you could never — he'd had his say before we got in. You could never get out of that place.

Sally was successful in being sent home on parole to her mother.

> When me mother were living, that's when I got out, when there were committees. There were a big board all round table. 'What do you want to go out for?' 'Where do you want to go?' They let me go but when me mother died I had to go back. Me brother wouldn't take me, he said there were nobody to look after me 'cos they were both working.

On another occasion her success was short lived:

I got out and stayed with me aunty and uncle in Brighton. I were doing shopping, looking after five children, I were getting on very nice. But some neighbours wrote t' doctor that they were not relatives to me. So I had to go back again. (I felt) lousy when they told me I were going back there again. It must be three times I've been back there.

In addition to admission and discharge, the Board of Control were responsible for monitoring standards.

The Institution is constantly visited by members of the Board, when patients are seen and any real or imagined grievances are carefully listened to and considered. Although as is but natural, there are frequent requests for discharge, the inmates are on the whole as contented as would be expected, given the necessarily indefinite conditions of their detention.

The Board of Control made a formal visit annually to inspect the hospital. The above quotation suggests that there may have been a prejudice on the part of its members to view the institution in a favourable light. Be that as it may, the institution prepared itself in advance of these visits as Sally recalls.

They'd see how we used to be treated. We used to put soap on the villas and put a lovely towel on. And toilet rolls in the 'toilet. We never used to get toilet rolls hardly. Everything were so spotless, I said, 'This isn't how we have it you know' — oh that nurse could have given me something. I said, 'Oh you've come when it's all nice!' They'd make us look nice an' all.

Sally's account is corroborated by Grace:

It used to make me laugh at The Park. They were so deceitful at The Park. Why couldn't they have told the truth when they used to have the Board of Control that came round every year. Well, they used to get all 'bathrooms and put towels on baths. Well, we never had towels. And they used to put soap in 'sinks. We never even saw soap! They did all that, just to make an impression. Anyway, I told 'em about it. I said, 'You know it's not always like this, it's only because you've come'

The Park and the Board of Control colluded with each other effectively, for the Board always gave The Park a satisfactory report!

2

'Colonies: Homely and Simple'

The Ideal System

> It is not possible to estimate the saving in the number of defective children that would have been born of the feeble-minded women who have been kept from child-bearing by segregation and supervision provided under the Mental Deficiency Acts. (Local Authority Mental Deficiency Committee Annual Report 1932)

The first institution to be set up by the local authority was opened in 1917 and was intended to be a 'Girls' Training Home' providing a 'protected homelife' for twenty-eight 'improvable defective' girls over fourteen years of age. The priority given to setting up accommodation for young women described as 'medium or high grade' is evident throughout the early development of institutions in this locality. This clearly reflects the authorities' prejudice that these women were more immoral than and 'twice as prolific' as other women and thus in danger of 'reproducing their own kind'. All those admitted in the first year were said to be in 'moral danger'.

Whilst undergoing training in domestic occupations, laundry work and needlework, some of these women would provide valuable services for the larger colony institution that was to be set up by the council two years later.

> The Park is admirably situated for the purpose of a colony in a secluded position. The land generally is pleasantly wooded, slopes gently to the south and is surrounded on all sides by a fine belt of trees affording both protection and privacy. (Official opening brochures 1932 and 1941)

Doris, who was admitted in 1936 at the age of twenty-nine, can remember The Park before it became a colony:

> I'd been to The Park many times before I'd come there. Used to come down to that mansion did the ladies and carriages and horses. It was all fields. Me uncle used to take me in the Park, it were lovely. Just for an afternoon out, go round country places.

As soon as the First World War came to an end, the county council was able to finance the development of a 'Colony for Mental Defectives'. With this purpose in mind the council bought The Park Hall with 175 acres of land. The eighteenth-century Italianate Mansion was arranged so as to accommodate eighty-seven patients; females of any age and boys under fourteen. There was also a small cottage near the Hall which was made into a 'hostel' for one resident staff and ten 'feeble-minded' men who were sent out to work.

Despite the spaciousness described in the brochure published for the colony's official opening in 1920, it seems that conditions were already overcrowded by the time nine-year-old Joe was admitted in 1921:

> It were just the Hall then, lads at one side, girls at 'other. I didn't have a bed — they put me on 'floor. I were laid on floor all night. It were bloody uncomfortable that! It was 'cos they had no more beds.

The founder of Britain's first colony, Mary Dendy[1], believed that the colony system would be more humane and efficient than the old one-block asylums and workhouses. The colonisation of so-called 'inferior peoples' was already a well-established and popular British policy at this time. The 'village' layout was to include all the basic essentials for housing, occupational and recreational needs. The colony would be as self-sufficient as possible with a central administration block surrounded by pavilion homes or villas for patients and various amenities such as kitchens, a laundry, workshops, recreation hall and a farm. For the local council there was the advantage of allowing the addition of buildings as funds became available.

In 1924, The Park Colony's first villa was opened to accommodate seventy patients. The Girls Training Home was closed and its patients and staff moved over to the new building. Further buildings were not added until 1930. However, with pressure to detain more people, the local authority had to rent two buildings in the late 1920s to help relieve overcrowding. 'The Orchards' opened as a separate institution to the colony. Similar to the Girls Training Home, it accommodate forty young women occupied in domestic activities within The Orchards and The Park Colony.

> It were just a big house. It had been a proper house but they made it into what they called The Orchards. It were very nice, old-fashioned but it were lovely. Plenty of fruit, plenty of strawberries. There were hens and their own eggs. There were fruit, apple garden, potato garden. It were nice there. (Grace)

---

[1] Dendy, M., Appendix in C. P. Lapage *Feeble-mindedness in Children of School Age* Manchester University Publication No. 13, 2nd edition, 1920

Elizabeth was one of the first patients admitted shortly after having an illegitimate baby. The Orchards operated a less restricted form of care than the colony as Elizabeth tells in her account.

> We used to have more fun at that big house than anywhere else. We used to have a walk and we used to go into the Abbey, have a walk round there. Do our shopping round there.

Oakwood was (and still is) a large imposing building, in those days standing right on the colony boundary. It was adapted to house sixty-four men. David came to the colony in 1929 at seventeen years of age. He was moved to Oakwood after having stayed in the men's hostel.

> 13s (the first pavilion home) were up when I came. They were planning how to put other villas up. I used to live in the Oakwood. There were some other lads used to live there, a lad what got mad. Frank he used to live in Oakwood with me.

Frank was fifteen years old when he was brought to the colony in 1932:

> I came straight up here to the mansion. I saw matron, then I got took over to Oakwood. We walked across with one o' nurses. I was wondering what that place was. It was all woods, thick woods. Woods on that drive coming down. A good few lived down there. I wanted to go back out!

Oakwood closed in 1932 when the first major extensions to the colony had been completed.

In 1928 a limited competition had been held to find the best and most economical plan for a colony to house one thousand patients. A Board of Control Report on colonies (1932) stated that with this many patients there was a danger of people losing their identity and the colony its 'community spirit'. The villa system was to be the means of preventing this.

By 1930 work to complete six villas and a school for The Park Colony had begun. The villas were officially opened in 1932 and were described as having been 'designed on the simplest lines, strict economy in construction and cost of maintenance being the dominant consideration.' Another dominant consideration, of course, was to arrange the new buildings so as to keep the majority of male and female patients separate. The most important task was to segregate certified women from mainstream society and female villas were given priority. No new villas had been built for the men at this stage but on the side designated for them was the hostel that had been enlarged and the 1924 villa.

To be cost effective, villas must not be too small: but they were also not to be so large (i.e. over sixty patients) as to destroy 'any impression of homeliness' (1932 Report). Accordingly the adult villas at The Park were originally designed to accommodate sixty patients each, the children's villas housed fifty and those for people with more severe physical and mental handicaps forty patients each. By today's standards, it would be hard to imagine the dreadfully cramped and barren conditions as at all homely; in most villas there was less than a foot between the beds and sixty (often more) people were to eat and relax all together in large dining/day rooms. Yet despite this, on some villas, patients and staff were able to make the best of things and create a generally congenial atmosphere:

> There were wooden chairs and pipes and a big, old-fashioned fireplace. It were all girls on that villa when I first came. It used to be all friendly 'n that. (Grace)

As Doris points out, the nurses in charge were important determinants of the character of each villa:

> It were nice over on villa 4, it in't now but it used to be the best. There used to be a Sister there, she was right tall. She was nice. Those two villas used to be the best. There were all different nurses on every villa, some were nicer than others.

The presence of open fires is clearly remembered and seems to have helped to make the villas feel cosier:

> And they had ordinary fireplaces, ordinary fires. We had to put coal in. They used to bring loads of coal outside in 'yard and shovel it all in, coal, coke all of it. Fires in every room. It used to be warm and nice. We had them wire netting guards. (Grace)

Though it was perhaps not so warm for patients who were not so assertive or who had mobility difficulties:

> They used to have proper fires, black coal. And they (the other girls) all used to stand behind the fire with their hands behind their back 'cos they all used to freeze to death! (There was) a guard so nobody won't get burnt, 'specially the children on 10s. (Margaret)

It is also clear that the so-called 'high-grade' villas, especially on the

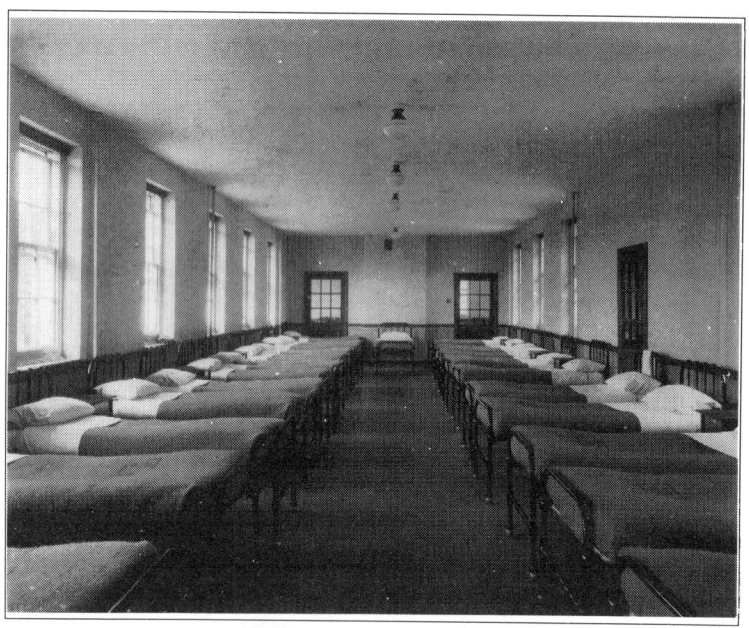

2.1 'There will be no justification for the expenditure of large sums of money.' Dormitory accommodation, circa 1940.

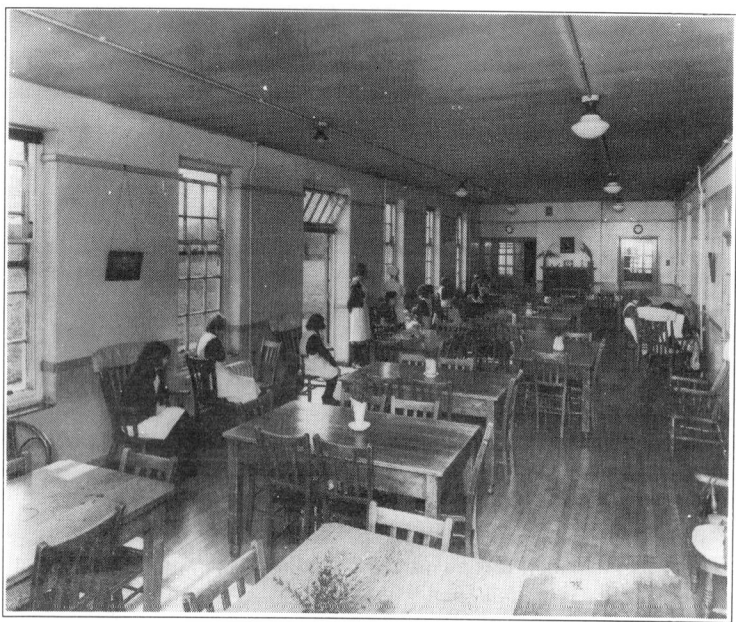

2.2 'There were wooden chairs and pipes and a big old-fashioned fireplace.' Day room on a villa for sixty 'high grade' female patients.

women's side, had a more homely atmosphere than the others. As well as being generally more socially skilled, the more able patients were on the whole treated in a more humane way; after all, their help and co-operation was much needed by staff:

> It was my home was villa 4 and villa 5. On villa 4 it were 'high grade'. The Sister what was very, very nice and we got it so it were who you could live with and who you could work with. Villa 6 was 'low grade'. Some of them on 'villas were in them things, tied up their hands, strait-jackets. Sometimes girls on villa 6. They used to do 'cos they used to tear everything. (Grace)

> I were working outside, not on the hospital. It were a high-grade villa. There were high-grade patients, them that worked out. You could go out on your own and that. (Frank)

Each of the villas had 'two side-rooms that were for punishments.' There were also specially built punishment villas with more side-rooms. The people with the most severe handicaps were not only offensively referred to as 'lowest grade' but as the 1932 report suggested they were to be 'situated apart from all other homes and away from the main approaches to the colony'. A great sense of shame was associated with these people and consequently they were placed well out of sight of everyone whether within the colony or without.

Because of her severe physical handicaps, from the age of six Margaret spent her childhood on one of these villas and remembers feeling cut off from the rest of the colony:

> Felt awful, lonely.

Apart from contact with 'working girls' and other 'helper' patients, Margaret got to meet others, 'only if we went for a walk with staff'. In the early days these patients do not seem to have been provided with wheelchairs. George came to the colony in 1936 and, as his friend recalls, he had the determination to withstand sore knees in order to get about the colony, 'on his knees, crawl upon his knees. Anywhere he goes, walk on his knees.' The 'low-grade' homes were also the only villas to have both males and females as there was little danger that these patients might enjoy sexual relationships.

With these new buildings the authorities now prided themselves on being able to reorganise and classify the patients. For many patients this entailed being moved over to different parts of the colony.

> They started building 13 (the first villa) and got it done. Girls were still in

'Hall and later they started to build some more (villas) round the park. All the lads were pushed out o' Hall and shoved in them. Women lived in 'mansion and they built villas on the other side o' park and they put all the girls into them. (Joe)

The colony's Annual Report for 1932 stated that 'the patients (were) transferred to villas appropriate to their needs and condition.' In fact, there were only two villas for adult men. Frank was one of the patients transferred and seems to have found life in the new villa as unstimulating as at Oakwood commenting that there 'weren't too much doing there.'

Official records dated two years earlier had expressed the intention of transferring all the patients out of the Hall when the new villas were built so that it could be used as the central administrative block and staff residence. However, it seems the demand for patient accommodation may have prevented this from occurring for some time. Grace was seventeen years old when she was admitted to The Park in 1932.

> When I went there, I were in the front hall a good long while. I slept in a little bedroom. (There were) about thirteen or fourteen of us. There were nice beds, we were comfortable. It were all girls. Then we used to have a shop and a big bakery where you go for your bread, next to 'mansion at back. (Grace)

Having since spent many years on the large villa dormitories, it is not surprising that in looking back Grace recalls that the bedroom for fourteen people in the mansion was small. Joe and Frank also remember women patients living in the Hall at this time and Frank explains:

> It were them that worked in the kitchens that lived in the mansion. The old kitchen down the yard there.

The mansion, like many other old buildings, is reputed to have its own ghost. With its surrounding trees and maze of passages it is not hard to see why some of the women who lived in the mansion claimed they had sighted the 'White Lady'.

> Used to see a bloomin' white lady walking up 'steps. It were quite true. They wouldn't believe us. She used to come down there with a long white skirt on and a veil over her head. (Doris)

Within a few years yet more accommodation was being planned for female 'defectives'; this time a large house, Abbey Grange, was purchased so as to provide an annexe for thirty-one 'medium-grade adolescent girls'.

I says, 'Where are you taking me?' They said, 'You're going down to Abbey Grange.' Belongs to here, but it were worse than it is now. It was as bad as it was up here in 'olden days. It were there somebody reported me saying I was after fellas or fellas after me and I got sent back up here. (Elizabeth)

Unlike the First World War which delayed developments, the approach of the Second World War accelerated proposals to complete the colony as accommodation was needed for emergency medical services. The new extensions were finished in 1940 and officially opened a year later by the Princess Royal. As well as providing more patient accommodation, the new buildings included various amenities to increase the self-sufficiency of the colony. The recreation hall was equipped to seat 600, rendering the use of outside facilities for social and religious activities no longer necessary. The colony became more and more insular and cut off from the local community as it grew. A new kitchen, bakery and general stores block were built at the back of the Hall along with a boiler house. Improvements to the Hall itself had to be postponed. The school had been enlarged and a hospital villa for patients who were ill was built with separate male and female wings. There were also new, and of course separate, workshops for men and women patients. The planners had taken precautions to prevent any contact whatsoever between men and women patients, the new laundry 'planned and sited so as to permit male staff to deliver and collect the washing without traversing the female and children's area of the site.'

The accommodation provided for staff and patients sharply reflected the strict hierarchy of the colony. A large, detached house with extensive gardens outside the main site had been built for the Medical Superintendent and, for the Chief Male Nurse, there was a new lodge house by the colony entrance. The new nurses' home included self-contained suites for senior officers and bed-sitting rooms for sub-officers. The opening brochure proudly states that seventy nurses could be accommodated 'each with their own separate bedroom having its built-in wardrobe and lavatory basin (h & c).' What a contrast to the villas where the same number of patients were to share one large dormitory, two bathrooms and two toilets! Old photographs further highlight the difference between patient and staff accommodation. The nurses' home has comfortable armchairs and settees with cushions and rugs. There were no such comforts for the patients. It also seems that villas intended to house patients classed as 'high grade' were larger than the others.

Once again the authorities hoped the new accommodation would enable patients of a similar 'mental and physical maturity' to be housed together. Because of the Second World War, however, all the new villas were used for wounded British soldiers and German prisoners. So despite the new buildings, there was still lack of space and accommodation.

Although the complete colony could now accommodate 841 patients, only 550 were resident. The presence of British and German soldiers could never be mentioned in official documents. A local general hospital had to be used as a 'place of safety' whilst the colony was unable to take new admissions. Elsie's move to another part of the colony during the war was likely to be the experience of many at this time:

> I came down here in t' war. In t' wartime it were all bare this place.

The colony was obviously at bursting point and patients probably more cramped than ever. Nevertheless, the authorities officially denied any overcrowding on villas and insisted that 'with few exceptions inmates of any one villa are of approximately the same level of intelligence and age.'

Whether or not this was actually true at that time (1941), in 1946 ten-year-old Tom found himself placed on an adult male villa when he first came to the colony:

> I was a bit frightened when I first walked into (villa) 13. (There were) some old people, some very old people.

Conditions had got so bad by this time that the authority's Report for 1946 disclosed:

> In recent years the lack of accommodation has led to the concentration of more aggressive, undisciplined children and youths among the admissions. They have shown a refractiveness to discipline which has been aggravated by the shortage of staff and of suitable accommodation.

An example of how the unbearably inadequate and overcrowded conditions affected patients is shown in Tom's statement concerning bathtimes on one of the children's villas.

> You used to fight over baths! There were only one bath. One bath for all of us! (Fifty children)

Ernest also tells of how tempers exploded on the villas:

> The villas used to get very noisy. There used to be quite a lot of quarrelling

and fighting. There used to be the quarrelsome kind and any little thing that came up... It used to go to such an extent that damage was done either to one or both patients concerned. It got to the extent that one of the injured ones would have to go to hospital for some form of treatment, so bad one was in need of operation. So I didn't get involved in any way in what was happening, kept out of their way.

The colony accommodation was further restricted when The Orchards was closed in 1946, reported as being in a dilapidated state. The soldiers had vacated at least one of the villas by this time and some of the women from the Orchards were placed there.

In 1948 the colony and Abbey Grange were re-named as hospitals to be run by the newly formed National Health Service, but conditions remained the same. Seven of the eight villas used by the soldiers had been returned but four of these were without staff or being repaired. The overcrowding not only jeopardised patients' mental well-being, but also their physical health. Reports at this time mention outbreaks of infections such as Sonne Dysentery and infantile paralysis due to overcrowding on villas.

(It was) too crowded, that's why they used to make more villas. There weren't much room in the bedroom. It weren't healthy to be too close together! (Grace)

The continuous removal of patients to different villas must have been a very unsettling experience for people already starved of security. At least some were able to resign themselves to the institution's reasons for being moved around:

As you got older you got moved. (Grace)

Some of the moves were felt to be beneficial:

I got told it was getting too crowded. I thought it were all right. It was a bit better. I was happy. I didn't like being on where it was too crowded. (Horace)

(I wanted to move) because it smelt! (Enid)

In 1950, alterations were made to the mansion to provide administrative offices and senior staff residences. Official reports mention the problem of staff shortages and even providing transport from bus and tram stops failed to attract new staff or prevent the high turnover.

By 1955, there were about 850 patients resident at the colony. One villa originally intended for seventy patients housed seventy-nine with only three staff. Even with the 'correct' number of patients, the purpose-built villas were found to be extremely inadequate for the accommodation and care of people with mental and physical handicaps. Conditions were quite simply appalling for patients and staff alike.

> They used to call it 'mucky colony', the patients, 'cos nobody liked it. They used to get told off and shut up. (Margaret)

It is no wonder that conditions had become so bad since policy-makers had largely neglected the plight of institutions such as The Park since their implementation. The Mental Health Act 1959 was the first major revision of the law relating to people with a mental handicap since the 1913 Act. The degrading certification procedure was dispensed with and 'mental deficiency' was replaced by the, many would say equally derogatory, term 'mental subnormality'. Most of the patients were now classed as voluntary and technically free to leave should they wish. Some of the more able did so, with little or no preparation for life in the community. For the hospital the Act did not improve conditions and the loss of these patients was disastrous: they had been unpaid staff, workers whose labour was essential.

When fifty-year-old Enid was admitted the year following the new laws, her impressions testified to the prevailing conditions.

> It stunk! It still smells. (Sharing bedroom?) Noisy, Lily cries all night.

After fifty years of having been looked after by her parents, Enid was very unhappy with villa life. She remained in The Park for twenty-five years until her death there in 1988.

Perhaps the best feature of The Park is the beautiful grounds which are a credit to the work of gardening staff and patients. The 1932 Report on colonies emphasised the importance of having attractive grounds, both to encourage parents to give consent for detention more readily and to be appreciated by patients. Although many patients may well have valued the beauty of the grounds, generally they were only allowed to enjoy them actively on special occasions such as Sports Day. Until a few years ago there were 'Keep off the Grass' notices. However, as this rhyme, whose words were sung to a popular tune, illustrates, neither the grounds nor living rent free compensated for being shut away:

Rockin', rollin', ridin',
Out of The Park Gates

All the staff are after me
Can't you hear me say:

'Oh, I'm fed up of The Park
Walking round all day'
Lovely ground,
Trees all round
There I have to stay!'

Home I want to go
I don't want to stay
Where there is no pay
Where all the nurses
Are bullying us so.

'Oh, I'm fed up of The Park
I've no rent to pay,
Lovely ground,
Trees all round,
There I have to stay!' (Grace and Sally)

3

'What Have I Come To?'

First Impressions

> My grandfather didn't say where I was going. He told me that I was going somewhere but he didn't say where. That's what got me, he didn't say where. If he'd 've said where I were going I expect I didn't want to come!
>
> Fetched me straight up here to the Mansion. Frightened I were. 'What's this place?' I saw the Matron, then I went over t' Oakwood, that big building over there.
>
> I walked across wi' one o' charge nurses. I were wondering what that place were. It were all woods, big woods on this big drive coming down. I felt awful! I'd rather been outside than be in a place like this! Couldn't go out, not outside. Inside at night. I wanted to go back out!

Frank's parents were dead and he had been living with his grandfather when he was brought to the colony in 1931, aged fifteen. He has lived there for more than fifty-eight years and has 'wanted to go back out' ever since. Frank's account expresses the fear and confusion that must have been felt by most people, whatever the level of their comprehension, who experience the trauma of being 'put away' in a large, depersonalising institution. Henry was only six years old when he was brought to the colony in 1931:

> I thought it was a home first time. It looked strange! A little bit nervous, a bit frightened when you first go in. You don't know anybody till you get used to them.

Like Frank, others also bitterly remember being deceived and the sense of having been betrayed and rejected by their families:

> He (Mr Grey) came and said I were going home. Instead of taking me home he took me to another hospital and I never saw me mother or father. They wouldn't get me home; they wouldn't have me in for holidays. (Elizabeth)

> Me mother put me there 'cos I wouldn't do as I were told. I don't think she wanted me to get on; didn't want me to be free or anything. She wanted me to be locked away. (Grace)

(I felt) awful, upset. What did me mother put me in here for? (Sally)

Of course, not everybody was willingly renounced by their families; illness, old age or poverty often gave families little choice but to hand people over to the authorities. Life at the colony was very different to the ordinary, albeit poverty-stricken, life-style to which most people were accustomed. Even those with severely restricting handicaps would probably find their quality of life diminished.

Admission was marked by a set of procedures which totally disregarded personal dignity and underlined the 'special' way of life people were entering. On admission new patients had to be examined by the colony doctor (after having already been medically assessed twice just prior to admission):

> I went t' Town Hall to one doctor. Then I had to go the Mansion doctors there. There was a doctor you had to see him before you went to all 'villas. (Doris)

Many, like Tom and George, were bathed and put to bed before the doctor saw them:

> A bath and bed (was the first thing that happened). (George)

> That's right I remember that. Had a bath, then 'doctor came. Been tested, got tested just to see if everything's all right. Just put thing on and do like doctors do. Then I got back up again and got dressed again. (Tom)

Following people into the institution were the certification papers that documented and emphasised only the worst aspects of people's lives and behaviour. These damning and personal details were, of course, fully available to senior and administrative staff and no doubt influenced the welcome people received. True or not, inmates were unable to escape these character references; they would be recalled for years to come to justify continued detention.

The system demanded that people put their previous existence behind them to take on the new identity of colony patient. According to the rules, any personal possessions were to be 'handed over at the earliest opportunity for custody':

> I never did see 'em, if I did take any with me. I weren't meant to see 'em! (Grace)

> Took your money or whatever, if you had any. You had to take what they wanted you to have. (Frank)

Perhaps the most obvious manifestation of this new status was the confiscation of people's clothing to be replaced with the typically drab institutional wear:

> We couldn't take any clothes and I could've taken a lot of me clothes. But I couldn't take 'em — no! There was a dress, a flowered dress, and that's what I had on to come in. But I didn't see it any more. I don't know where it went. My father gave a lot of my things away, coats and good clothes.
> We'd only 'uniform all the same. White aprons and hats all the same and black stockings and boots. Sometimes shoes and no underclothes like we have now. We had striped knickers. An old-fashioned skirt all week and then at the weekend these old dresses, dark green dresses. We'd only one for the weekend, dark green with white aprons. We hadn't anything else! (Doris)

The clothing issued to the young women destined to be 'working girls' is remembered as being particularly uniform-like and degrading:

> I were dressed nice when I came up to The Park. Never see them no more. They take 'em away and they won't tell you where they were. Put them striped things on. The way we were dressed, I used to think it were disgusting! Long frocks and boots on. No shoes, we weren't allowed to wear shoes. Well your knickers were just the same as them striped things butchers wear. Bloomin' old-fashioned corsets like aprons what fastened at the back. We looked awful! Your 'names' on a piece of tape – number 4, ward so-'n-so. Mine were number three. (Grace)

> We couldn't wear us own clothes, we had to wear theirs. We wore striped dresses, black stockings, striped skirts and all institutional clothes. Everything with that hospital on it — with your name on it. You've to wear it whether you liked it or not. I used to do what they told me to — put them on! (Elizabeth)

The men and children did not fare much better:

> They took mine away from me, the clothes I used to have. Put 'em away somewhere, I didn't see 'em again. I had to wear theirs. Old clothes! We had what they give you. What they got from the sewing room. What wi' colony on; all marked, 'The Park Colony', inside 'collar. They were patched. On 'trousers at front and at 'back. Girls used to do that in 'sewing room. Underclothes — they were marked 'n all. (Frank)

> You had to wear their clothes. Used to be old rags! They weren't like they are now. I were in shorts, short trousers. Then boiler suits and hobnailed boots for bricklaying. Used to count them all up with their names on the back of the collar, numbers on hats. (Henry)

With the Board of Control urging managers to 'ensure clothing is not of unduly expensive quality and not discarded until past repair', it is hardly surprising that patients' clothing is repeatedly referred to as old, old-fashioned and patched by those who had to wear it.

Part of the reason for marking clothes was to minimise 'sharing'. Nevertheless, garments would certainly have been passed on when patients died or left the colony and were probably communal in the 'lower-grade' villas and in times of acute overcrowding. Staff today recall that there were communal underwear stores on each villa until very recently. However, it was clear to some of the inmates that there were other reasons besides those of economy and practicality for issuing clothing so obviously marked as institutional:

> You couldn't run away in them clothes! My mother used to change mine in 'graveyard. (Grace)

> What wi' colony on; all marked, 'The Park Colony', inside 'collar. In case you run away. (Frank)

> If they thought you'd wear your own, they thought you'd run away! (Sally)

Institutional clothing was characteristically colourless, well-worn, old-fashioned, often ill-fitting and the same, come rain or shine. Inmates were aware that their clothes marked them as different or inferior.

> Going to church three abreast in them bloomin' boots! We looked awful. (Frank)

Adult colony patients were also required to have standard haircuts. For women with long hair, this simply added to the distress of being admitted:

> I were as clean as anything when I first went up there. They didn't even comb me hair and they do do. They cut it and I know that! And that made me worse still. I had it long, you see, right blondie long. And all you could wear were one clip. You couldn't even put it in curlers. You had to do what you were told! I never thought I'd get out. (Grace)

For able-bodied newcomers, becoming a colony patient also meant work and some were assigned to duties on the very first day:

> Dr Black saw me the first day. He just asked me how old I were and I told him. He said, 'Do you like working?' I says, 'Yes'. 'We'll see about getting you a job in the recreation hall.' Sweeping up, polishing the floor, that were

the first day I went! (Horace)

The first two weeks at the colony were known as the 'settling-in period' and during this time, new patients were not allowed visitors:

> You'd got to get settled before they let you have any visitors. You'd got to get settled first for a fortnight. I think it did good 'cos you'd realise that ... if they let you have visitors you might just run out with them. That's what they thought. I used to cry when me mother went home! (Grace)

How could new patients be expected to get over the trauma of being removed to such a strange, new way of life within two weeks?

> When I first came I thought, 'Oh God, what have I come to?' That was the first thing that got into my head — what have I come to? It were frightening for me. I just say, 'What's up with this place?' when I first came and you couldn't talk to any o' lads. 'Oh God!' I said to one o' lasses, 'Is this how you've been brought up — without talking t' lads?' She says, 'It's been like that ever since I've been here! You'll get used to it when you've been a bit.' I thought, 'Oh God, I want to get away from here!' And I've been here ever since! (Elizabeth)

> I was so heartbroken when I first went up there! I cried a lot. I didn't like it but you couldn't do nothing else! I wouldn't bother with nobody. I were poorly for a long while. (Grace)

Most of the villas were kept locked and, one way or another, the system forced inmates to accept the institutional regime, but some could not accept that this was to be their home for the rest of their lives.

> I was a bit fed up. Well, you wouldn't like to be locked up all your life! You would not! It were taking you all your time to bear it. (Grace)

Admission to large institutions inevitably involved the loss of individuality and privacy. Inmates were handled in large blocks; collectively regimented and conducting all their daily activities in the presence of other patients and staff:

> You could have no privacy on 'villas. It did used to get on my nerves having a nurse sat with you all the time! (Elizabeth)

> Didn't like people watching you all the blessed time! It were like a bloomin' prison! (Grace)

> When we went anywhere, we had to have staff, two staff, one at 'back and

one at 'front! (Elizabeth)

Staff were looking to see, keeping their eye on them to see if they were up to mischief. (Margaret)

You couldn't go t' bathroom on your own. Oh no! There were staff with you all the time! I used to give 'em looks when I went! (Grace)

One lavatory for 'patients. They had doors but no locks on. I used to be scared many a time, be frightened that they'd come in! (Sally)

As in prisons, letters were automatically read.

Patients' mail was censored in the Chief Male Nurse's Office.

All letters, either out-going or in-coming to them, must go through the office of the Principal Nursing Officer. Members of staff are forbidden to accept any for postage or delivery elsewhere. (Hospital Rules in 1960s)

This was not because the recipients may have been unable to read: it was simply part of the system of absolute control.

You could have your letters, when they'd read 'em. They used to go t' office. It weren't nice but you couldn't say nowt 'cos if you said anything you got punished. So I wasn't going to get punished over it. (Grace)

There was little comfort to be had under such large-scale communal living where conditions caused much unhappiness, anger and frustration:

The villas used to get very noisy. There used to be quite a lot of quarrelling and fighting. (Ernest)

When they had these violent ones, they used to wreck it (the villa) up! There was iron chairs and iron tables. They were awful to sit on. But if they had decent furniture, couches and chairs, the ones that played up bad used to rip them up in tempers. That were no enjoyment for us. They spoilt it for us. I know they couldn't help it but that was a bit too much! (Sally)

Even basic equipment for personal grooming and hygiene, such as bath towels and combs, was communal for most patients:

Combs, used to share wi' others. If you got one of your own it were all right. (Frank)

Any personal possessions that the patients were able to obtain were almost impossible to keep because of lack of privacy and personal space.

> I used to have a little case for all me clothing and that. I had some books — drawing books and that — tracing books. Somebody took 'em. (Henry)

The more privileged patients had bedside lockers, but these could not provide any safekeeping as, despite the name, they did not lock! Clothes were also in danger of being taken since these were also to be kept in the lockers:

> They were always pinching! (Enid)

> If you had a book, others would take it, if you put 'em in your locker! It was awful, wicked; flippin' terrible it were! (Frank)

> When we took 'em (clothes) off, we had like a locker to put 'em in. I didn't like the lockers what they used to have, I didn't like 'em! Couldn't lock 'em — anybody could take your clothes! It were a bloody nonsense, clothes in them days — anybody could take anybody's clothes. (Frank)

The only way patients could have their things kept safe was to put them in a cupboard on the villa which only staff had access to:

> Had a case or summat like that. There was a cupboard downstairs used to put it in. You had to ask for it. (Frank)

Such conditions were bound to cause friction; some patients developed obsessive attachments to collections of material that would otherwise be seen as rubbish, others vented their anger on vulnerable patients:

> If they had birthday parties, if they didn't get the prize in that parcel passing, they started carrying on. One . . . she was right violent, if she didn't get what she wanted, take it out on 'others. (Grace)

A strict and punitive system put all patients under physical threat. To maintain order and discipline, natural reactions to stressful circumstances had to be suppressed. Patients were kept in line by the ever-present threat of punishment; either the withdrawal of privileges or more severe measures.

Nine-year-old Joe arrive at the colony in the year after its official opening. His first impressions recall the brutality that this system yielded:

(It was) awful! I didn't care for 'people that were in it such as 'doctors and nurses. I didn't like them at all! I didn't like any of them hardly. They were hitting the other people, knocking them about. It weren't nice at all. Once of them, the nurses, put a person in a bath of cold water. That weren't any good for them!

Although admitted forty years later, Enid's first impressions of life at The Park were much the same as Joe's:

They were bossy, they hit! They used to do it for nothing! (Enid)

Dependent patients were in danger of physical harm not only from staff who were careless, tired, resentful or violent, but also from the able 'helper' patients venting similar emotions.

There were ones who made their feelings felt by being rough with the less fortunate ones; roughly handling them in the way they went about the job they were meant to do. (Ernest)

There were even times when incontinent patients were blamed or punished for their lack of control:

Staff used to get mad with them. They used to say, 'What've you done that for, you dirty thing!' (Grace)

Although people did not ask (or even want) to be institutionalised, the 'care' they received was very much seen as being provided by the charity and goodwill of the state. Naturally this attitude was conveyed to patients, obliging them to be grateful, especially for any 'treats' they received:

I'm not going to call it . . . it were very good. (Grace)

We always said grace. That's what I liked. We used to say 'thank you' for what we got. It was a very nice thing. (Grace)

It weren't a case of choosing (presents), you had to be content with whatever you received which I was happy about. I used to always receive something that was of some use to me. (Ernest)

The National Insurance people were 'only ones that sent them (presents) and to other places. Well they do that, National Insurance, don't they. I'm glad they do. (Henry)

They used to give us (a party) on us birthday — give us a do. I won't say they didn't give us them things like that 'cos they did. (Elizabeth)

In things that we as adults take completely for granted such as food, clothes, leisure pursuits, and bedtimes, the colony patients had very little or no choice at all. For example, with all meals, patients had to 'have either what had been sent or nothing.' On some villas, patients did not even have the choice to leave unwanted food:

> If we didn't eat it, they'd save it for your supper. You had to eat it and eat it and eat it till it were gone! We daredn't leave anything, them days. We daredn't even say to staff, 'I don't want this.' You daredn't be rude! (Margaret)

On the one hand the inmates were completely controlled by the system, and on the other, they suffered severe neglect. Far from being alleviated, people's handicaps were increased by restrictions that stifled personal development and autonomy. Intentionally or not, the system literally degraded the people it labelled as 'mental defectives'; the system reflected society's attitude that they were sub-human, unworthy outcasts of society. At its most benign, the system viewed patients as perpetual children and treated them accordingly:

> Mentally defective persons are never likely to attain a normal stage of intelligence or reach a minimum standard of citizenship. They are in reality infants and should be regarded as such.[1]

> They treat us like children not women! It were awful. I were glad when I came away! (Elizabeth)

---

[1] Wormald, J and Wormald, S. *A Guide to the Mental Deficiency Act 1913* King and Son, 1914

4

'They Treat Us Like Children!'
Routines, Rules and Regulations

> You'd all have to be up for half-past six or seven.
> We couldn't wear us own clothes.
> We weren't allowed to talk to any boys.
> Staff used to be in 'bathroom with you.
> When we went anywhere we had to have staff.

A certain amount of routines, rules and regulations is necessary in all our lives but in the large institutions these 'three Rs' completely dominated and regulated every aspect of life. As well as being essential for the smooth running of an overcrowded and understaffed institution, they were an integral part of the 'control and supervision' of patients thought to be morally at risk. In practice all patients and most staff were governed by a strict institutional regime.

Each weekday at the colony was much like the next, with an early start to the day:

> Well, we used to get up at half-past six. Breakfast at eight and then we had to start work then. (Doris)

In the colony's worst days some patients were awakened at 5 a.m. so the villa night nurse could have them ready by the time the day staff come on duty. Little wonder, then, that they had to have the more able-bodied residents helping out.

> We used to get up about half-past six to get them (other patients) ready. Give them their breakfast first then get one after. They (staff) appreciated it. (Horace)

> Had to be up at half-past six to get dressed and washed and all that. The routine was the same as usual, take the 'wanderers' for their breakfast. They wouldn't let us sleep in! (Henry)

When getting dressed, patients had no choice in what they could wear:

> You've to wear what they put out! You've to wear it whether you liked it or

not. I used to do what they told me to do, put them on! (Elizabeth)

Breakfast was usually bread and butter with a cup of tea or sometimes porridge.

Two slices of bread — couldn't have extra! (Grace)

Porridge were like I don't know what! (Elizabeth)

Had just a drink at home. (Joe)

Joe was lucky enough to get a full cooked breakfast at the farm he worked on outside the colony. Only a small minority of patients worked outside the colony. After breakfast many of the more able patients went to school or work in other parts of the colony whilst the rest would remain on their villas. For these latter people daily life was even more limited with no purposeful activities to help the hours pass and very little or no opportunity to experience surroundings other than the villa they lived on.

Just stopped in 'place — 13s and just sit about and think about a lot of things. (Tom)

This seems particularly ironic since this group of people, who must have included those with more severe handicaps, were probably the ones most in need of a stimulating environment. Frank sums up how he felt about life on the villa:

There weren't too much going on there. Every day were just, well, boring!

Margaret describes some of the activities she was able to do on the villa once she left school:

Didn't used to go to work yet, just stayed on the villa. Just talk to somebody and do jigsaws and games or dominoes. You know, crayon books and drawing and things.

Patients working in the colony and the colony schoolchildren returned to their villas for lunch.

We went back t' villas for lunch. Stews and dumplings. (Horace)

After lunch patients either returned to work or school or stayed on the villas. For the evening meal, patients 'used to have just ordinary tea, not cooked'. Grace was said before meals. As with everything else, patients were to be grateful for what they received. However, after a day of physically demanding work, even the women who appreciated saying grace felt the bread and butter tea was inadequate:

> Well, what's two slices of bread to a girl that's working like . . . (Grace)

One patient felt so dissatisfied about this after working hard outside that he spoke out about it:

> Didn't get a hot meal then. Same as usual, bread and butter. I complained about it. I said, 'I'm not going back home till I get a proper meal. We're not working out in this cold weather and that's how you think about it . . . going back for a cold meal! (Henry)

Health services spend less on food in mental handicap hospitals than in general or psychiatric hospitals. The daily allowances of food for each patient and those for the staff in 1933 is available in the records (*see* table overleaf). The difference between allowances for staff and those for patients, e.g. butter instead of margarine, and the addition of fish, marmalade, jam and fruit, reflects the position of patients in the colony. The lack of a hot meal after midday for both residents and staff must have saved the management money in both food and heating costs.

There was, of course, little choice and many people remember the food as being poor.

> You couldn't pick, you got to have what you get! I didn't care for 'apple crumble, it was awful! People having diarrhoea with it. You didn't want to bite it! (Henry)

> Many times the food was off; affected by change in weather conditions. Just leave it — there was nothing replaced it. If we did leave anything because it had been affected by change in weather conditions, it was just a case of leaving what was there and doing without the meal, otherwise enjoyed so much. In many ways it has changed for the better. I enjoy all my meals now more than I used to then. (Ernest)

> Used to have to carry all the dinners from the kitchen to villas. They didn't have motor cars like they have now going round with it. I wish there had've been. I can make me own Yorkshire puddings better than what they can! There again, I never saw bloomin' Yorkshire puddings. Bloomin' rice pudding was like water. You couldn't have extra. (Grace)

However, some people do remember food as being better in both

The Park Colony – Sample of Typical Dietary Allowances 1933

	Breakfast			Dinner			Tea			Supper	
	Patients (oz. per head)		Staff (oz. per head)		Patients (oz. per head)		Staff (oz. per head)		Patients (oz. per head)		Staff (oz. per head)
Cocoa	$\frac{1}{4}$	Tea or coffee	$\frac{1}{2}$	Stewed meat	6	Roast mutton	6	Tea	$\frac{1}{4}$	Tea	$\frac{1}{4}$	Coffee
Porridge	2	Porridge	2	Vegetables	4	Potatoes	6	Bread	5	Bread	4	Bread
Syrup	1	Milk or syrup	2	Potatoes	6	Vegetables	4	Margarine	$\frac{1}{2}$	Butter	$\frac{1}{2}$	Butter
Bread	4	Fish or brawn	5	Milk pudding	$\frac{1}{2}$ pint	Rice pudding	$\frac{1}{2}$ pint	Cake	2	Jam	1	Fruit or cheese	$1\frac{1}{2}$
Butter	$\frac{1}{2}$	Butter	$\frac{1}{4}$			Bread	2	Syrup	1	Fish paste	2	
		Marmalade	1									

Notes: 1. The meat allowance is weighed uncooked. 2. Bread is allowed ad lib. 3. Morning lunch supplied to children consisting of $\frac{1}{4}$ pint of fresh milk. 4. Milk or treacle supplied with porridge. 5. From May to September stewed or fresh fruit or bacon or brawn to be supplied instead of porridge. 6. Hot cooked meals are not to be supplied for staff suppers. 7. An issue of fresh fruit, an egg, and a ration of liver to be given to children once a week.

quality and quantity in the early days of the colony: Mabel, for example:

> One thing that was best about it, was we had good meals. Good food. The food was good. It isn't now — it's awful stuff now. Awful. I don't call it food. (Mabel)

Grace, at Abbey Grange, remembers good food in the old days.

> It was beautiful. We got lovely apple puddings, apple pies and everything. It were beautiful down there. The Orchards was just the same. They'd bake all our own bread and cakes for us, all our own teacakes. The bread were too thick for me at The Park. It was ever so thick, bread. I don't like thick bread. (Grace)

> We had good meals. The food was good, it isn't now. They used to cook pork and beef and real boiled hams and tongues. We used to do our own potatoes. They used to make them sponge puddings with treacle and jam. You don't see anything like that on villas now. A lot nicer stuff then, it was beautiful! (Doris)

> Years ago, the food wasn't so bad. (Margaret)

Perhaps when the colony was smaller in the 1920s and 1930s and the farm with its market garden, chickens and pigs was flourishing, the quality of food was better. Opinions of the quality at present are distinctly unfavourable!

The evening routine, as in the morning, had to fit in with staff hours of duty and thus most patients:

> Used to have to be in bed before 'night nurse came on at eight o'clock. (Elizabeth)

After tea, some patients would help nurses clear up and start to get 'those who couldn't help themselves' ready for bed. Patients described as 'lowest grade' would have tea, a bath (or 'a good strip wash') and then bed. George remembers being put to bed at six o'clock when he lived on the children's villas and at seven o'clock when he got older.

On certain nights of the week there were some routine leisure activities, usually in the recreation hall:

> There were no tellies then, no tellies at all, so the only nights we went 'out' were (some) Saturday nights for concerts, Monday nights for Guides and Thursday nights for 'pictures. (Joe)

These events were subject to very specific routines and regulations:

'constant watchfulness' is stressed in the hospital rules.

> Patients were lined up outside their villas. Those that wanted to go were checked in number so that they knew, when it was time for them to come back after the show, that the same number that went down were returned. All the male patients used to sit on one side of the hall and the female patients on the opposite side. (Ernest)

On the evenings when 'there weren't anything going off' the patients who were not busy helping the nurses or being put to bed early might listen to the radio, do some knitting and sewing or chat to nurses and other residents. The patients who went to bed later than eight o'clock were either those favoured by staff or those working late around the colony.

> We put 'others to bed at eight o'clock. Then we went downstairs and stopped to listen t' wireless. We were called the helpers.

> We used to have to be in bed before 'night nurse came on at eight o'clock. Nurse used to say, 'When so-n-so comes off duty, you can come down and keep me company.' She'd whisper so others wouldn't hear her and report her. (Elizabeth)

> I remember they used to let us in and we used to go straight upstairs 'cos we'd had our supper. Same wi' working at the nurses' home, we'd come home at half-past nine and go straight upstairs. (Grace)

> Male patients had to be in bed by 8.00 p.m., except for a few on villa 15 who were allowed up a little longer. (Ernest)

At the weekend, the morning routine was the same even though most patients did not have work or school to go to.

> They wouldn't let you stay in bed like you do here at weekends. You'd all have to be up for half-past six or seven o'clock unless you took poorly. (Frank)

> We got up about seven thirty and went to bed at nine o'clock at the latest. It was at the weekend as well. (David)

At the weekend patients were to wear their 'best' clothes:

> An old-fashioned skirt all week and then at the weekend those old dresses, dark green dresses. We'd only one for the weekend, dark green with white aprons. We hadn't anything else! (Grace)

Saturdays must have been much like any other day on the villa for patients who did not go to school or work. Patients normally 'out' at work during the week also found themselves villa-bound on Saturdays. Naturally this became tedious, week in, week out, year after year:

> I was just a bit fed up. How would you like to look out of the window on a Saturday and couldn't go out anywhere?! You wouldn't like it!! (Sally)

In the evening, the monotony of the day was sometimes broken by regular picture shows or concerts that were put on in the recreation hall. Such events were accompanied by the usual segregation and head counting procedures:

> They used to have some concert parties coming up to entertain us on a Saturday night in the recreation hall. (Ernest)

On Sundays, the recreation hall fulfilled its other main function, as a place for religious services. Church-going was an institutional activity that was very important to many of the patients and was one of the routines in which they gladly co-operated.

> I used to go to church. Used to be in 'choir; used to know all the songs going I did! (Joe)

> We used to go to 'chapel. I still do. I've been going since I was about ten years old and now I'm sixty-two. I keep up to my rules! (Henry)

Some patients remember going to the local church and picture-house outside the colony before the recreation hall was built in 1941. Only the most capable and able-bodied patients were allowed the opportunity to worship in the local church, and then only if they passed Matron's inspection as they were counted before leaving the colony:

> We used to go to the village church. Used to line up on 'top drive for inspection before you went to church with Matron. See that you were clean, if your boots were clean and your hair done and clothes were all right. If they weren't you got sent back into 'villa. (Frank)

No doubt Matron and her staff were especially vigilant to ensure patients' appearance and behaviour were a credit to the institution. Jewish patients were visited by a Rabbi who made special arrangements for them to observe their religious festivals. Some services were also held in villas for those unable or not allowed to attend the local church and recreation hall once it was built.

We used to have church on Sunday afternoon on villa 5 and have service. (Joan)

Some of the routine events occurred on a weekly or monthly basis. One of these events most looked forward to by some was visiting day:

> We didn't half look forward to visiting day. Once a month, then they changed it so people could come at night. (Mother visited) every month, never missed. She was little and small but she never missed me; buy me frocks, buy me fruit. Two o'clock when they opened it (villa) up. They (visitors) had to stay outside — queue up. They weren't allowed in till the door was open. Then they used to go in the dining-room for visitors. Sat there till four. They were sat with you all 'time at the table. (Grace)

As with everything else, visiting times were strictly regulated to a set day, time and place. Parents who could not manage to come on that day and wanted to arrange another time were informed in writing:
'It is necessary to adhere strictly to the regular visiting days.'

It was also a strict rule that visitors under the age of fourteen were not allowed.

> Only us mothers and fathers were allowed to come in and see us. If your sister came to see us, they had to look through the window! (Margaret)

Even though some aspects of patients' hygiene and health were not part of the colony's daily regime, nevertheless they were dealt with at specific times and with yet more routines and regulations. The bathtime routine was especially governed by rules and regulations, warranting its own rule book, 'a copy of which must be posted in every bathroom, (and) must be strictly adhered to at all times.'

> You never got bathed on your own, you'd got staff with us and you had to wait in queues. You weren't allowed to touch the baths yourself. Taps were took off 'cos they were like taps you had to screw on and when you'd had your bath they took 'em away. Or else some people would kill themselves, drown themselves. (Grace)

Patients were usually bathed once a week. On some villas all the patients were bathed on the same day. With just two baths (and usually two staff) per villa this could take two whole days and, according to one nursing assistant who was working in the colony in the 1950s, was like a sheep dip.

My villa bathed weekly, mostly at the weekend when we didn't have anywhere to go. We would go in alphabetical order. (Ernest)

Used to get a bath Mondays and there were no more till 'Monday after. There were two baths in one bathroom. The water weren't always too warm, like on the cold side. They used to bath us. All the taps on 'baths used to be with keys. He had a key for 'hot tap and a key for 'cold tap. They used to wait outside the door, others who wanted a bath. After they'd bathed you, they used to dry you and then book you down that you had had a bath and cleaned your nails. (Joe)

Patients were bathed by staff regardless of any ability to do so themselves.

(It was) not like it is now; I'm put in the bath now and I just have someone to do the parts I can't manage myself and then left to carry on myself until I'm finished. (Ernest)

A local barber came to give the male patients a regular shave and 'short, back and sides' haircut:

There used to be a barber at The Park. He used to have one of those cut-throats. He was a good barber; he used to be a barber in his own shop. He'd shave you nearly every week when you got told to come. He used to let you help him. (Henry)

As Ernest points out, patients then 'didn't have a lot of choice'.

He'd just do it for you. Sometimes they did it as they thought it ought to be. We didn't have a lot of choice in one thing or another as it is at the present time! It was rather annoying! (Ernest)

Staff said, 'You need a haircut,' so I had it cut. (Horace)

The nurses used to cut the women's hair. Old photographs show most of the young women with uniform 'bobbed' haircuts.

They used to cut it. I used to get them curlers, 'dinkies', and curl it under. (Elizabeth)

They used to cut your hair, the nurses. Didn't go to a hairdressers then. They used to do it all right. (Doris)

Two women who spent their childhood on the 'lowest grade' villas remember having long hair:

Me and Joan had right lovely long hair and had lovely bows in us hair, lovely! (Margaret)

The colony, with its rules and regulations for everything, clearly regarded daily dental care as unimportant and impracticable in the institution. There was no regular routine for cleaning teeth. So, like the majority of the general population at this time, most patients had poor teeth and eventually many would have to have them all pulled out. The Annual Report of 1951 shows that there were just over 300 inspections, of which 250 resulted in extractions. There were only 74 conservative treatments recorded.

> The dentist would notify staff who were in charge on the villa when they were to see you. You would be seen in alphabetical order. We would go, to villa 3 (hospital villa) where the dentist was. If it was a case of having any trouble with teeth, you would have them taken out! I didn't have a lot of trouble with mine fortunately! (Ernest)

> Went t' dentists, villa 3. Don't mention it, they pulled all my teeth out! They had to have permission from me parents to have 'em out. (Tom)

> I used to have me proper teeth and then I had them all pulled out. I don't know why; 'cos they were bad or . . . The villa staff told me when I were gonna have them out. Then after a while when me mouth cleared up, then it were false ones. (Margaret)

> Dentist up there came to pull your teeth out. Horrible were 'dentist, used to have your teeth out! (Sally)

In the overcrowded conditions, there were inevitably periodic outbreaks of infections and infestations.

> I were poorly once, I had dysentery. Sometimes they used to find crabs; shave all down there off. Put you to bed then. Didn't want anybody that were infectious, didn't want anybody else to get it. Somebody passed it on to be by scratching. I got rid of it. (Henry)

Many patients, especially those who were bedridden and incontinent, suffered badly from skin rashes and infections.

Although part of the justification for special institutions such as The Park was to provide better and more specialised medical care, relatively recent reports, such as the annual reports of the National Development Team, have shown that in fact patients received poorer primary health care and had less access to specialists. Because they were classed as mentally defective and lived in an institution, patients' needs for specialist treatment outside the colony were either ignored or treated as only of secondary importance. When Frank, who was already blind in one eye, was referred to a surgeon for the removal of a cataract in his other eye, the surgeon questioned whether, since he was an institutionalised patient, potential blindness would be a very great defect for him and whether he would be likely to benefit from an improvement in vision! Because the authorities did not consider him suitable for discharge and he was unable to read and write, surgery was not considered advisable at that time. Frank did eventually have an operation ten years later but it proved unsuccessful.

For the most part, patients seem only to have been given routine medical examinations when they were admitted and when their detention orders were due for renewal. However, the Medical Superintendent did carry out daily rounds of the colony villas:

> Dr Black used to come round every morning — never missed. (Grace)

Patients only saw him personally for the more serious illnesses and 'offences'. The individual attention and medical care given to patients when they were quite poorly does, however, stand out in people's memories.

> He (Dr Black) looked after me when I had arthritis. It were him that found I'd got it. He were very good to me. (There was) a German doctor, he were lovely. He were out on to them villas before you knew where you were. (Grace)

> Used to keep awake when you had dysentery, Dr Black. Used to come round and see you when you were poorly and keep you in bed for so many days. And they died from dysentery, people, didn't they? (Frank)

The doctors generally seem to have been more at home with 'proper doctoring', i.e. treating physical symptoms rather than psychological ones. Seriously ill or infectious patients would be taken to the hospital villa where at one time a doctor and his wife lived. Elizabeth remembers this doctor taking good care of her when she had bronchitis.

> I were at The Orchards; I took poorly and I had to come back here (the main colony). Matron and Dr Black come for me and I was spewing me heart up. When I got there, I went over to villa 3. Doctor and his wife used to be there. He didn't half look after me. If they hadn't 've looked after me I would've been a goner! (Elizabeth)

Certain physical functions such as bowel movements, menstruation and epileptic seizures were all monitored in the villas' daily report books. Patients were routinely subjected to enemas and medicines to regulate their bowels. One nurse recalls that all epileptic patients were given weekly enemas: constipation is believed to increase the likelihood of a seizure. Patients well remember having to take the white medicine.

> We used to take that white medicine. Cleaned your bowels. (David)

> White mixture, that white stuff. Same as that kaolin stuff. Toilet again; used to drive me round the bend! (Tom)

> Every Tuesday morning was called 'whitewash day'. We used to line up for it. It made people incontinent. (Sally)

Patients were expected to conform to the institutional routine, body and soul!

5

'You Did Anything Wrong — God Help You!'

Ensuring Obedience and Respect

People who were certified and admitted to large institutions were necessarily stripped of the support provided by social relationships and the rhythm of life at home with their family and friends. On admission they were required to adapt and accept a totally different enclosed and alien world. Many recounted the fear and apprehension they felt during their first few days and weeks. The Park colony was a total institution: it attempted to provide for a whole variety of education, work and residential needs through a single bureaucratic system which was isolated from the rest of society. Such a system required the suppression of individuality, although since The Park was a colony and not a prison, its intent was benevolent rather than punitive. Its aims were to develop good work habits and a sense of achievement, whilst at the same time operating under conditions of strict supervision and control. The ethos was primarily that of confinement and control at minimum cost.

The institution regulated everything and in this respect The Park was little different from the sort of total institution described by Goffman in 1968.[1]

> The patient's life is regulated and ordered according to a disciplinarian system developed for the management by a small staff of a large number of involuntary inmates. In the system the attendant is likely to be the key staff person, informing the patient of the privileges and rewards that are to regulate his life and arranging for the medical authority for such privileges and punishments.

To run efficiently, any large institution not only has to have rules but also has to have ways of ensuring adherence to these rules. This philosophy is summarised in the 1949 Park Annual Report as follows:

> The payment of conduct and industry rewards continued to encourage habits of regular work and good conduct. The rewards were graded according to the

[1] Goffman, E. *Asylums: Essays on the Social Situation of Mental Patients and other Inmates* Pelican, 1968

mental state of the patient and the type of work performed and were reviewed regularly by the medical staff. The money was spent on purchases of sweets and tobacco or were saved for purchases made on shopping expeditions to town.

Trustworthy patients were granted increased freedom within the colony and were later allowed to make unescorted visits to town. The hope of securing these privileges stimulates good conduct in the more intelligent and stable patients.

Rules and regulations were designed for the smooth, efficient running of the institution: they did not allow for individual self-expression nor did they permit some basic human rights to be respected. The institution controlled everything, including contact with parents and relatives and the world outside.

Leave is a privilege which is earned by obedience to the regulations.

This system was vividly recalled by Ernest:

Patients had to be careful how they behaved in their work and on the villa or wherever they were 'cos there was strict staff in those days and any offence, they used to be up before one of the senior doctors. In the case of first offences, they were warned of the serious nature of the offence and what would happen if that or anything like it was repeated. Then they were placed before the doctor and they lost all their privileges for a certain length of time. As far as privileges were concerned, (they) used to be going to films and concerts and in the hospital grounds, recreation hall and money included.

The hospital rules euphemistically referred to the necessity of watchfulness at all times as demanding 'a high standard of tactful guidance by the nurses'. What constitutes 'tactful guidance' is not specified but staff were no doubt aided in their work by the payment of conduct money. The colony operated a system of conduct money payable each week to patients. The purpose of this money was to encourage obedience to the rules. In practice the operation of this system went well beyond the rules; it was intended to develop and maintain a respectful attitude to authority.

You know being really rude to staff and swearing. They'd go in front of Matron and Dr Black and all them. They used to get into right trouble. They really got into bother then. . . They couldn't go t' pictures or anything like that, concerts, where I was saying we go, until they learnt to behave themselves. (Margaret)

Put them to bed just for swearing. (Grace)

You got your money stopped for two months or three months. You didn't get a penny. For being cheeky or anything like that. Sometimes you'd stick up for yourself like mad, you were on your own! (Grace)

Obedience and respect were the order of the day.

They were strict though. They used to tell them to put them to bed without supper if they didn't do as they were told. They used to try and take them upstairs to bed, make sure they get in and take their clothes away.

Staff had their own way of dealing with minor problems. Problems such as incontinence created extra work and could lead to punishment even when a person's physical handicaps prevented them from having control of their bladder and bowels. Grace tried to forestall trouble on her villa.

I used to tell 'em who to excuse and who not to excuse. Well there were some that couldn't help themselves. I told her which ones had to go to t' toilet. They had to keep changing them 'cos they kept being wet. When they got bathed, they changed their clothes 'n that. If they couldn't get there quick enough they used to do it on 'floor. Staff used to get mad with them. They used to say, 'What've you done that for, you dirty thing!' (Grace)

Margaret, who is unable to walk and has little control over much of her body, has first-hand experience of such treatment.

If you were bursting to go somewhere and you wet yourself, you know like with me, you got punished. Say you were in a wheelchair and you couldn't talk to tell them, you still got punished — couldn't go out, couldn't see your visitors.

Margaret also recalls staff's attempts to get her to eat all her meals.

Shall I tell you something else — if you leave your food, you know what they used to do? If you didn't eat your dinner — leave it for your tea. And if you didn't eat it for your tea, you had it for your supper and if you didn't eat it for your supper you had it for your next meal. It's true!

Joe, seething with a sense of injustice, recalled with relish his one successful attempt to get his own back on a member of staff who was trying to force him to do something that he did not want to do, namely scrub the floor. Because he refused, he was given 'the treatment'.

I said, you do it yourself. So they grabbed me and got a bucket (of cold water) and poured it on top of your head to make you do as you were told.

So I thought to myself, 'Right, I'll get my own back' and I did it on her.
I got sent to Dr Black. He said, 'What's happening here?'
I said, 'She threw that cold water on top of me.' He said, 'Yes, why?'
'She wanted me to scrub the floor, so she threw a bucket of water on me and I got a bucket of water and poured it on top of her.'
He said, 'You shouldn't do that.'
I said, 'She threw it at me first so I threw it back.'
He didn't know what to say himself.
I slung the bucket down then said, 'She can clean up any mess herself.'
They couldn't do owt. What could they do? (Joe)

Punishment varied according to the severity of the offence. The most often employed was the control of money, 'they'd stop your money'. Restraint and physical punishments were frequently recalled as consequences for more serious offences such as any attempt to meet a member of the opposite sex or for absconding from the colony. Often both restraint and physical punishment were combined. A period of being locked in a side-room was often followed by some penance such as being made to scrub floors in pyjamas or underwear.

If you got caught doing summat to a girl, they used to lock you in a side-room. They used to run away did some of them and they had to bring 'em back and put 'em in a side-room. And scrubbing — used to have shorts. Same wi' girls. They used to do the same on the female side. We used to go round and see girls just in their knickers scrubbing floors. Villa 8 was their locking-up villa. (Horace)

John, he went on to villa 17, locked up in the side-rooms with no clothes on. (Horace)

They punish them. Put 'em in the side-room until they behaved. It were awful. They didn't use to have pyjamas on then. They used to have short pants on. That's what they had. (Henry)

They put you in pyjamas for scrubbing and that. You would be put in pyjamas. (Frank)

They used to make you scrub from one end to t' other. And if you didn't do it proper, you had to do it over. Sometimes, if we didn't do it, we didn't get anything to eat. They once put me in bed without any tea. (Sally)

Absconding was the direst of offences. However, this illegal freedom was very easily obtained.

It were easy. Go into 'wood down there and you were away. Just wandered about. Out for a few days. Sleep anywhere. Caught up with by the police — brought me back. Used to be awful when you were fetched back here. (Frank)

I used to sneak out from open bedroom window — where you come down 'stone steps. I used to open 'window that opened at bottom. We used to get out at night. (Grace)

Grace remembered one desperate young woman's attempts to escape:

There were one girl there on villa 6. She hadn't been on long. She were a little devil — used to get straight up the chimney and get out. Used to go to Town Hall, black as ever. 'Cos doors used to be locked all time, it made people worse. (Grace)

Such an offence merited removal to the punishment villa, if you didn't already live there. Of course, there were separate punishment villas for men and women. In each, confinement in the side-room was combined with fatigues like scrubbing the floor. For men, the punishment villa was villa 17, for women, it was villa 8.

Villa 17 was different from other villas because that was where patients who tried to get away was taken. It was known as the punishment villa. They had side-rooms where patients were taken if they'd done anything seriously wrong, trying to abscond from the hospital. (Ernest)

17s it were, when they used big punishments. They were scrubbing floors and carrying sand, bags of sand and if they dropped them there is somebody behind them to tell them to pick them up and keep carrying them. And when they scrubbed the floors, they had to scrub it again, keep doing it all the time. That's why they got tired. They used to be in pyjamas and they used to have a dressing-gown on. (David)

They had some that run away. Put them on villa 17 in t' side-room for punishment. It's like a room you get locked in all the time, you can't get out. (Frank)

For Sally, life in the institution was unbearable: her attempts to escape the institution or life itself met with the same response:

I got a bit fed up of being there and I were missing me family. I used to do things to meself, cut meself 'cos I were depressed, being there so long. I used to break pot and slice it (arm and wrist) when I were in that room where they locked me. When they used to let me out sometimes, I used to go in 'toilet and smash a window and then do it, hurt meself. I hurt meself instead of hurting other people.
That's why I run off. The police were after me. I went out (on parole) with

another girl and while she were in 'shop, I run away.

Well, the police went to me brother's house and they said, 'We've got a warrant to see if your sister is here.' And they went upstairs to bedroom and everywhere and I weren't there. I took meself back to 'Abbey. Twice I went back by meself. They say if you go back on your own, they can't punish you. They did! When I got back, they put me in that room again! They gave me a cold bath, really cold.

They used to put me in a pen. A big square thing with all wire round. They put me in there all afternoon and it were snowing. And they took me back at night and put me straight back in that room. I think that's where I got me illness, arthritis. Then I was on floors in that room, no bed, just a mattress with strong ticking that cut your neck, that's all. And you had tin plates and basins. You weren't allowed any knives and forks, just a spoon.

(In a strait-jacket) they once had to do that 'cos I were doing that much to meself. They used to tie me so's I couldn't do it. (Sally)

Frank too tried hard to escape but was always brought back. When he was returned by the police, he explained to the doctor that he did not wish to stay in the colony.

He said I had to stop a bit longer. I've stopped here too long.

The punishment for Frank was the same, side-room and scrubbing the floor.

I've been put in there. . . I had to do floor and they were always at the back of you.

Conditions in side-rooms were bleak. The rooms were locked and were deprived of furnishings so as to prevent anyone from harming him or herself.

They were the punishment villa — where they gave you injections and put them in a padded room. They had no beds in, just a blanket on the floor. They used to lock them in there. (Grace)

They locked you up for punishment in a dark room with the shutter locked and door locked. All you'd to look at were four walls, for a month. You couldn't get any air. And you had nobody to talk to. It were just boring. All day for a month. I didn't even know where I were when I got out. Everything were different. (Sally)

When she put me in that room, she said, 'You're not going to see daylight where you're going, it'll be dark.' One nurse, she said, 'You ought to be there for six months, not a month!' (Sally)

Ensuring Obedience and Respect

Food was minimal.

> They got summat to eat, not much. Just got one potato, one bit of meat and what have you and one bit of pudding. They just had one meal a day. They didn't get nowt for tea, no breakfast, just a cup of tea. All they had was their dinner. (Horace)

> We had to bang on 'door for it. Sometimes you were lucky if you got any. And once, what they did, because I wouldn't eat it, they mixed it all up in a basin, put mixture in that makes you go to t' toilet and I couldn't eat it. See, I didn't feel hungry; I got so depressed, didn't want any. The white mixture that they gave me were terrible. It were horrible. That were just because I wouldn't eat. It were punishment. (Sally)

The urge to escape from what was in fact solitary confinement and the anger and resentment of those who were incarcerated simply led to a worsening of the physical conditions and a longer sentence. Sally told of one girl who managed to unscrew the lock with a spoon.

> They had one girl in there, got herself out wi' spoon. I don't know how she did it. When they went to her, they said, 'What have you been doing?' She said, 'Wouldn't you do the same if you were locked in here?' So they said, 'We're not as bad as you, you deserve all you get!'

Sally expressed her own feelings very strongly:

> Once I banged the door down. They had to put me in next one. Some of them used to sit down and bang with their feet on door. And one girl next to me, she were throwing 'chamber up and down. The chamber is what they wee in. They wouldn't let her out and all urine went all over!

Grace also recalls the conditions:

> The worst villa were villa 8. It was in a mess. Used to get drugs, bromide and all like that and locked in.
> When they had that bromide, it sent them mad. It was terrible, it sent them crazy.
> I used to cry when they used to say to me, 'Will you take this bread up to side-rooms.' I thought, 'Oh, the poor things.' On a bloomin' tin plate!

Estimates of how long people were kept in side-rooms varied from one day through to one week or as long as five or six weeks. Humiliation was an integral part of the enforcement system. However long the punishment may have lasted, in nearly all accounts mention is made of the practice of making offenders scrub floors in their pyjamas or underwear. One member of staff with some thirty years' service recalls the time when people were made to wash all the villa windows downstairs (more than twenty windows in all) both inside and out with cold water.

The simplest method of punishing the offender was just to remove him or her to the punishment villa. The congregation together of people who were consumed by rage, frustration and despair was often punishment enough without the need to have recourse to the side-room.

> Villa 8, it were a terrible villa with all the violence. They used to have some violent ones there. One big stout girl, she'd come out of Rampton. She used to go for all staff. That's why they were all frightened of her. (Sally)

Even in the security of a side-room, Sally was frightened.

> I used to be frightened that these patients would come in and grab me 'cos they wouldn't think twice. One next door to me, she were right violent. She used to go for staff. If she didn't get what she wanted, she'd take it out on others. That's why I kept me door shut so she couldn't get in. I used to wait while she went out, before I would come out.

Sometimes in this situation, the potential of violence could be channelled by staff towards those inmates they did not like or wished to punish. This, of course, they could do with impunity.

> She once got hold of me wi' hair and pulled me from one end t' other 'cos one of staff told her to do it. She (staff) couldn't do it herself, so she got her to do it. They were cruel. I thought she were going to kill me that afternoon. I were terrified. She (staff) were laughing like anything. (Sally)

It is unlikely that punishments such as these were officially sanctioned by the management. Institutions developed their own subcultures and the official systems of punishment operated by the superintendent and the matron may well have been supplemented by a more covert informal system of control operated by the attendants who were charged with the day-to-day care of the inmates.

Physical punishment such as beating and hitting inmates would have been expressly forbidden. However, it is not surprising perhaps that such punishment should have occurred. Frank remembers one charge nurse who would take people into his office, take a big stick out of the cupboard and belabour them.

> Used to get punishment. Used to hit them with a stick. They gave you a good hiding.

A system based on punishment and the fear of punishment is always a potential breeding-ground for violence and cruelty. Some people recall that particular members of staff operated their own system of sanctions.

> There were some nasty nurses what used to work there. We're only human but they were cruel! They used to bray people, sometimes for nothing. It were terrible, the poor lasses were really punished. (Grace)

> Mrs Brown, she used to be awful, her. You did anything wrong — God help you! (Grace)

> I didn't care for people that were in it such as nurses and doctors, I didn't like them at all. I didn't like any of them hardly. They were hitting other people — knocking them about. (Frank)

> It weren't nice at all. How I know, one of them, the nurses, put a person in a bath of cold water. That weren't any good for them. Some staff were going to chuck me in a bath of water with clothes on. So I ran at him and shoved him in instead. He didn't speak to me for months upon months. Then I got him sacked 'cos he was hitting others. (Joe)

Another way of coping with rebellious residents was to give them laxatives. Sally said that the 'white mixture' was added to her food as additional punishment when she was confined in a side-room. Such punishment was very effective: it is very difficult to cause problems for others if you have stomach-ache and have to run to the toilet frequently. Strong laxatives are physically debilitating and since their use was a routine part of the system, they were readily at hand. Again, they could be used with impunity since weekly laxatives were the lot of many residents in any case. In 1922, in his autobiographical account, Montague Lomax[2] drew attention to the cruel and dangerous practice of prescribing large quantities of Croton Oil as a punishment for rebellious inmates. Having taken some of this preparation himself, his experience of the effects was such that he made strenuous efforts to ban its use from the institution in which he worked. A laxative as powerful as Croton Oil may not have been used in The Park but the practice of using laxatives to control behaviour was well-established.

The more conventional medical treatments involved the use of drugs, often powerful and addictive sedatives such as paraldehyde.

> Some of them used to get needles to calm 'em down. They used to give me 'em. I were going mad. But I can't remember 'em giving me 'em, but they left me with a little lump in me bottom.

[2] Lomax, M. *The Experiences of an Asylum Doctor* George, Allen and Unwin, 1922

> They used to get bromide. I used to have it but they took me off it. They said it were no good for me. They said it could kill you in the end. I got so attached to it, I didn't want to come off. Sometimes when they wouldn't give me one, I wouldn't go to bed 'cos I got so attached to it. But they left me off it for a couple of nights. I didn't want it no more. (Sally)

Some residents coped with institutional life by taking care to avoid infringing any of the rules at all. Identifying with the system offered some protection.

> They didn't do owt to me and Horace, we kept ourselves clear. That's how we got out, not doing things like that. (Henry)

> I didn't do any running away. I don't, never have done. (Henry)

> They were towards us depending very much on how we behaved. For the most part, I got on all right with them. If we behaved well, we were treated well. If anything out of the ordinary which didn't do well, we were treated accordingly, according to the offence committed, whatever it was. (Ernest)

There was, inevitably, a certain amount of blaming the victim, even among the victims themselves.

> Oh yes, we wasn't made miserable, we wasn't even beated up unless we did it to us own selves. It was up to ourselves to behave. (Grace)

Joe found that the policy was to keep himself to himself.

> I just used to go about and keep me mouth shut.

Relatives and other people worried about the closure of institutions and the shortcomings of care in the community often picture the hospital or institutions as a safe place, a haven where people can be cared for and protected. Hospital scandals in the late 1960s raised public awareness of conditions and some improvements were made. There is now a belief that such things no longer happen. Whilst it may be true that some of the worst physical punishments do not now occur, punishment is an integral part of any institution. Like many people with a mental handicap, the people in this study are still subject to a system of rewards and punishment which we would find unacceptable for ourselves. Today people in institutions who infringe regulations for whatever reason are just as likely to have their privileges (such as visiting relatives or going to the cinema) curtailed, their drugs increased and/or their money withheld.

6

'I've Worked All Me Life Up Till Now'

Creating Useful Colonists

When The Park opened in 1920, no mention is made of a school although the institution did accommodate fifty-two female 'defectives' of any age and thirty-five 'defectives' under the age of fourteen. Mention is, however, made of a kindergarten: 'A qualified kindergarten mistress is also engaged in the work of training those patients who are able to benefit by the simpler forms of kindergarten occupations and this department has been equipped with suitable apparatus and models.'

Only two of the people covered by this study were admitted during the early period of the institution. One was over school age. The other, Joe, who was nine years old when he was admitted in 1921, is unable to remember this kindergarten.

> I can't remember. All I can remember, I sprained me ankle climbing over like some railings, climbing over into the park. I sprained me ankle and I couldn't walk. I just tried the gate they locked up, so I thought I'd try other way. I got over the railings, I were down and I couldn't get up any more then. Somebody came and took us home.

In 1922, the Board of Control reported after visiting The Park:

> We can see that no child with any manual capacity is overlooked.

The prevailing attitude of the Board of Control was that 'those whose mentality is of too low an order for any intellectual acquirement can often be taught to use their hands and so become of value later on in the routine of institutional life.' The local mental health committee endorsed this view: 'The training of the imbecile child produces a more self-dependent and self-reliant colonist and reduces the cost of maintenance.'

The 1931 extensions did include a school. By this time also The Park was able to provide accommodation for fifty children. The aims of education for the 'idiot and imbecile' classes accommodated in The

Park were considered by the Board of Control to be:

> in the experimental stage and the results to be achieved will depend largely on the application of suitable methods to the needs of each individual case. If commenced in early years, improvement in these damaged and shapeless lives can be achieved. The formation of habits of cleanliness, self-reliance and discipline will enable many of them at a later stage to perform useful work in the colony though it will be of an elementary kind.

Girls, in particular, would be taught to 'sweep, dust, clean, make beds, fold and iron clothes, clean boots, knives, spoons, etc.' Despite these educational principles, memories of The Park school seem to be on the whole happy ones. Joan remembers the school teaching money and games and Margaret recalls:

> When I got a bit older I learnt to write and that. They got me to learn how to — 'cos I couldn't talk when I first came — so they got me name down to talk. I only went to school in the morning, not the afternoon 'cos my mother used to come and see me every day then.
> We used to have singing and that first thing in school. Then we went into classes to do other things, like learning to do sewing and drawing and painting. When it was a nice day — used to go down the field and play in the sand, have buckets and spades and we used to go on swings and do all that.

A photograph of the school, taken in the 1940s, shows a class of well-behaved children being taught reading and writing. A teacher who taught there at that time recalled that the children 'were always keen to learn'. The children were neat and tidy and the school did not cater for those who were of the lowest grade. The principal function of the school was not literacy but the teaching of practical skills which would be of use to the colony. Housework and handicrafts figured largely in the curriculum. Henry, who was seven years old at the time he came to live at The Park, remembers being taught practical skills.

> We used to play games, learning to read and write, spelling and how to clean places up — how to wash windows, how to clean anything you can mention.

Some teachers were recalled as strict:

> She used to punish them. Put in 'corner with their hands on their heads. Put them on their knees until they do as they're told. Kneeling on a strong floor, they don't like that you see, it makes their knees sore. (Joe)

Those that were not admitted to The Park when they were children

Creating Useful Colonists

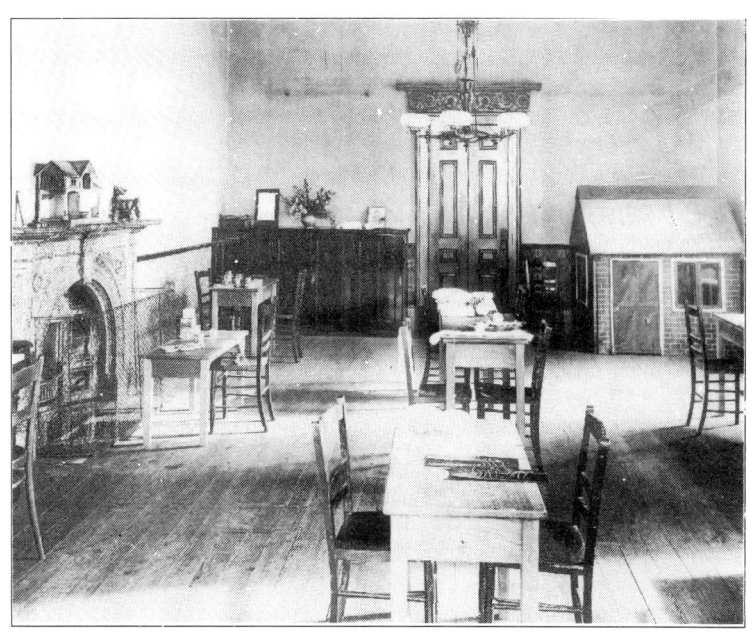

6.1 The first schoolroom, 1922 for: 'Those patients who are able to benefit by the simpler forms of kindergarten occupations.'

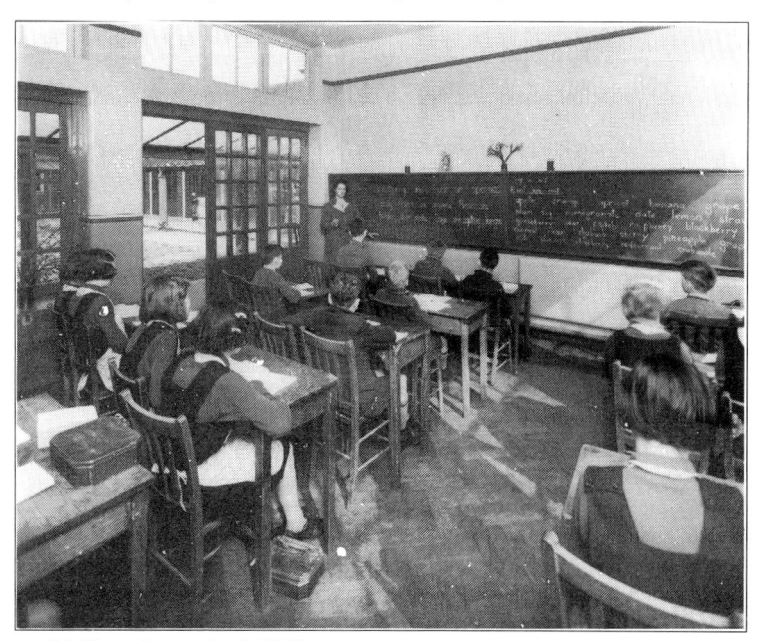

6.2 The colony school, 1947:
'Improving those damaged and shapeless lives.'

were sent to Junior Occupation Centres, if they were considered capable. The emphasis in these centres was similar to that of The Park school, that is, practical rather than academic.

> I've done a bit of reading and that. You had to do tailoring. (Joe)

> They didn't learn me much at all. Mother mostly learnt me to read and that. They didn't teach you very much at all. It were cleaning and all like that. It weren't like ordinary schools, but the school I went to before they did learn me reckoning up and all like that. (Grace)

David Barron[1] in his moving account of his own institutional life provided a sample time-table of his school week. This seems largely to have consisted of nursery activities and religion, interspersed with useful pursuits such as needlework and cleaning. The contrast between what was taught in schools for defective children and the questions asked of such children at the formal assessment for certification is noteworthy. In assessing mental deficiency, questions asked related to academic knowledge such as arithmetic, geography, grammar, general knowledge, reading and writing. The almost exclusive emphasis on practical skills in special education must have ensured for the colony a steady supply of able people who could readily be certified as 'feeble-minded'.

School was a preparation for work in the colony. There were considerable economic advantages accruing from such an arrangement.

> The cost of colonising the mentally defective compared with the cost of maintaining them in rate-aided Public Institutions or Hospitals not organised for their training and occupation, results in a considerable financial saving to the Local Authority.

Thus stated the brochure of the formal opening ceremony for the extensions to The Park in 1932. The cost of the institution would be kept as low as possible if inmates' labour could be maximised. The themes of work and preparation for work emerge strongly in the Annual Reports of the institution and of the Board of Control.

> Colonies, established and administered on practical and economic lines by means of proper utilisation of the labour of patients, appreciably reduce the cost of maintaining defectives in public institutions.

Work dominates the memories of those able-bodied residents who became, whether they would or not, part of the institution's

[1] Barron, D. *A Price to be Born* Published in 3 volumes 1981 –2, New Directions

cost-effective labour force. The rules of the institution in 1924 stated that:

> Bedmaking will be carried out by a special officer with the assistance of patients who will work under her supervision.
>
> Other patients will be allocated to various departments in the House, e.g. Laundry, Kitchen, Dormitories, etc., under the supervision of the officers in charge.
>
> The services of high-grade patients selected for the purpose may be used in assisting in the preparation of patients for bed, but such assistance should always be given under the supervision of the officer.

The use of patient labour is similar to that quoted in the 1929 Report to the Mental Deficiency Committee which classed 'colonists' as follows:

> The high-grade patients are the skilled workmen of the colony. . . the medium-grade are the labourers. . . the best of the lower-grade patients fetch and carry or do very simple work.

For female patients in The Park, this meant domestic work.

> In t' olden days I worked on a villa. Scrubbing on your hands and knees. I worked at night — till seven o'clock at night. Bathing them and putting them to bed — them being short-staffed. That's how they think I got me bad leg from when I used to do a lot of scrubbing every morning and every night. They didn't have vacuums or doings like that — like they have now. It were all kneeling. Mucky, dirty side-rooms to do. (Grace)

Scrubbing and polishing and bedmaking seem to have comprised the bulk of the work available for women in the colony in the 1920s and 1930s.

> We work. We had to scrub floors. There was nothing like there is now. We had to get down and scrub — polish it. . . Polish tables, chairs, clean windows, wash all paint. I used to wash all 'walls. Not high up on 'walls — doors and all bottom walls and bottom part of windows. (Doris)

In 1943, a laundry was built. It included provision for the employment of the less able residents whose job it was to hand-wash linen in stone troughs.

> That's where they used to do the towels out that were mucky. In the sink.

That was in the laundry. (Joe)

Although photographs of these rows of stone troughs exist, none of the women recall having to hand-wash clothes. Perhaps this is because most of them were classed as skilled work-women and therefore worked in the 'proper' laundry.

> Fold all sheets, blankets and things like that, and I used to pack them all up in right big baskets. I used to write it down who they belonged to. Nurses' home I used to do, doctors and mansion and all different wards. None of them could read and write that's why I did it. There was a woman there and she left. So she said, would I do it when she left? And I said, 'Yes, I would do it.' She said nobody else can read and write. I was a good worker in that laundry. I used to iron and press those things. They wanted me to go back once. (Doris)

According to the Annual Reports of the time, some 10,000 articles were laundered each week, the volume of work being valued at £8,500 per annum. The laundry was designed to employ fifteen female patients. Grace recalls working in this laundry, in the kitchens and in the nurses' home.

> I worked in the laundry. Sometimes I were on ironing and sometimes I were pulling sheets on the big machines. All of us got up early; half-past eight to 'laundry. Finish half-past five from 'laundry. I used to work in 'kitchen at night till half-past seven or eight o'clock. We used to cook potatoes and wash parsnips, 'cos staff used to have their supper at nurses' home. Then I worked at nurses' home. I liked it there. (Grace)

The pride Grace put in her work glows through her account of it.

> I worked on the villas. And I used to work where they had a sick room. And they (doctors) used to come every morning to say how beautiful it were: we used to keep it lovely!
>
> I used to have the most beautiful ward on villa 5 for sick people. I wish Dr Black were living just to see. It was beautiful. It used to shine like anything. I were a good worker up there. They only had to ask me to do it and I'd do it willingly.

She can also recall what it was like to be a 'working girl' helping on other villas. Her account underlines the physically hard work involved in keeping these wards clean and how upsetting she used to find working with very severely handicapped people.

> They had all wires up 'cos there's no freedom. 'Cos if they didn't, they'd go on the road — people that couldn't look after themselves. I used to go there

Creating Useful Colonists 73

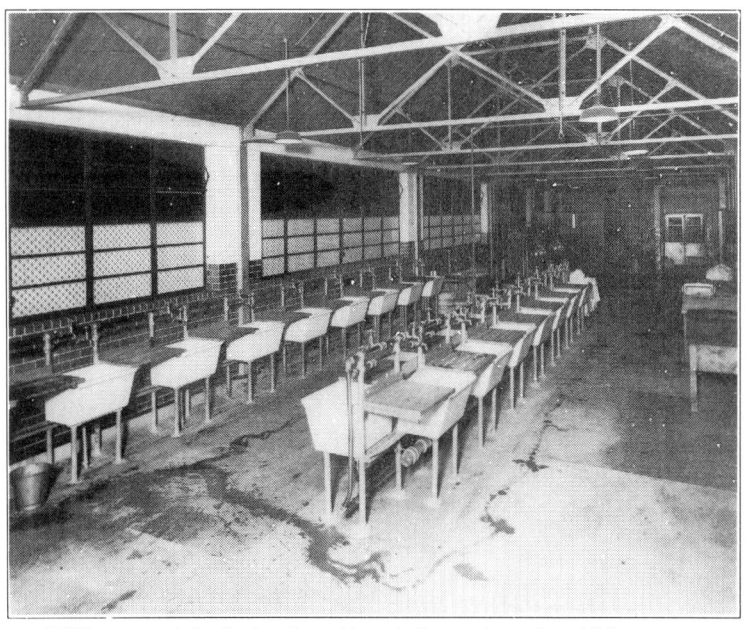

6.3 The stone sinks for hand-washing clothes and towels, which provided employment for less able female patients, 1943.

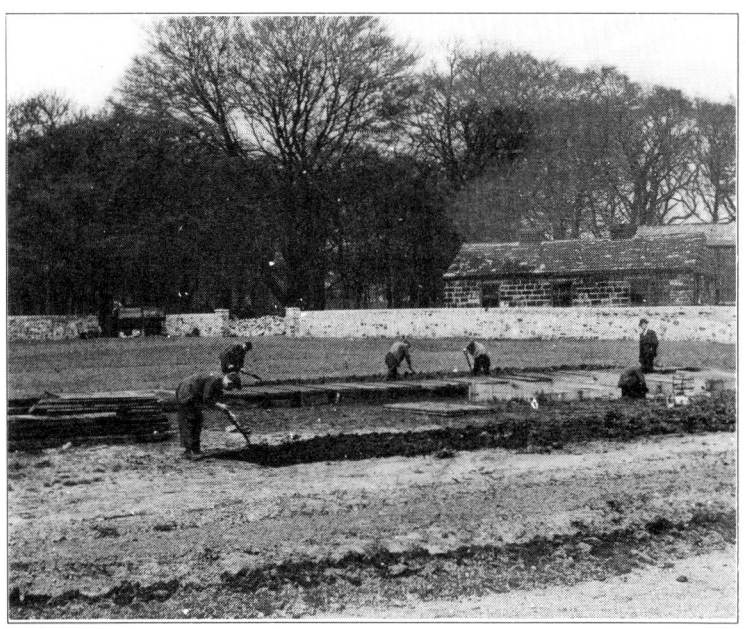

6.4 Preparing the ground for spring, circa 1935.
Note new boundary wall.

to work on a morning — I loved that job. It used to hurt me feelings but I used to love it.

We used to scrub those wooden floors with steel wool, used to get all in your hands. Your hands used to be sore. It were very hard work. I used to do it on 'villa in t' dining-room. It'd come up beautiful after but it were hard work! They made tea for you if you behaved yourself. But it were hard work! And we used to have to get coal in and coke until teatime. You had to put it on big shovels and shovel in into 'hole where it used to go. There were loads. And motor cars used to come wi' coke and you all had to go out, while it snowed an' all and you'd have to do it.

Nobody was ever lazy, 'cos you weren't allowed to be lazy. Had to do something. (Grace)

Because Margaret was unable to walk and, at this stage, unable to talk, she was one of the people the working girls looked after and she remembers them with affection.

They used to call them working girls. . . The working girls used to come every morning to make the beds. . . They used to say, 'Get that (wheelchair) through there you little devil — we're trying to make the beds' — I couldn't walk and there was Joan laughing all over the bed. 'Get back through there you little devil.' I used to get out of me wheelchair on me bottom and slide on the ground. (Margaret)

Working girls were also very useful when new staff started work: they used to show new staff the ropes and were recalled by some nurses as being more helpful and approachable than senior staff. Mr Tanner, a nurse appointed to the hospital just after the war, recalled that women did domestic duties or worked in the laundry, the nurses' home, the kitchens or the sewing room.

I used to work in the sewing room. We used to patch sheets for nurses. (Grace)

I used to fold up clothes in the laundry, and I worked in the big kitchen an' all. If you want to know — I did the potatoes. I also had to get the eyes out of the potatoes as well. (Voilet)

However, Grace found herself doing quite a different kind of job for a while:

At Abbey Grange, when I went there, I used to look after a right big boiler. Get up on a morning at half-past give, five o'clock sometimes, to get all the water ready for the girls to get washed. I were just coming out when they said, 'God, what's the matter with this girl?'

So nurse said, 'Oh, she's just been doing the boiler.'

'What, doing the boiler — a girl? That's a man's job not a girl's job. Tell her to come and get washed and come and see us.'

So I went to her and she said, 'You're not supposed to be in here dear. You're too bright to be in here.' (Grace)

These young women worked a very full week with more than an eight-hour day, yet none of them recalled being paid for the work that they did.

We never saw money. (Elsie)

We didn't get any money then. We'd not any money, we had to work for nothing. Work for nothing in them days. Then when it changed, you know the change-over, they started giving them money and he said, 'You can buy some clothes now of your own.' (Doris)

Nowt. I didn't get ha'penny — not ha'penny. But now it's all over — everybody gets a wage. When I worked in 'kitchen I didn't get ha'penny and in handicraft — I didn't get ha'penny. Not even a drink. But now it's all over. (Violet)

No, we didn't get money — not in them days. We got sweets. (Elsie)

When I worked in 'kitchen I didn't get a ha'penny, not even a drink. (Violet)

I don't know but I know that I didn't get a lot. We all complained but what can we do. Didn't get no more, just got the same. (Elizabeth)

Mr Tanner confirms that patients were paid or 'awarded' sixpence a week or a bar of chocolate. It may have been that the women were given chocolate and the men money for, like the women, the men worked long hours, but unlike them, most can remember being paid. When the colony first opened, the work available for the employment of 'ten feeble-minded men' was gardening, farm-work and boot repairing. Joe remembers working in a farm outside.

When I left school I used to be a market gardener. I used to go about... roots and stuff, cabbages, potatoes and cauliflowers, taking them round to houses. Bloke who used to go to market for some stuff like to take it out. There were two of them, two sons, I used to go with one one day then I used to go with the other. He was a coal worker. He used to carry coal — talk about heavy!

Used to start about nine in the morning and finished about seven or eight on a night. We had a break for lunch. He had like a shed up there, used to go in it. He had a table in and chairs in and kettle to mash tea and stuff.

After he was admitted to The Park, Joe was set to work on the farm.

> After that, I started working up at 'hospital then. Started from gardening, from gardening work I started with a pair of horses ploughing the fields. By, talk about it being heavy to swing about! My fingers were red hot, talk about sweat! As soon as I took me boots of, they started to smoke!

Henry arrived at The Park when the first extensions were being built and can remember building the boundary wall. According to Mr Tanner's account, this wall was made from stones dug from the grounds of the colony. Although Henry describes himself as a 'bricklayer', he was actually dressing and laying blocks of stone.

> I built that wall when I were fifteen. I taught meself (to lay stones). Can chip 'em out with a chisel. Used to kneel down on 'job, like a mat — a rubber mat — chip it and put stone on top of another stone and chip it that way... couldn't break heavy ones... I chipped it down to get it level. Then you grind it with a stone, make sure it's completely firm, that's the way I did it.

He can also remember being paid sixpence a week for his work and recalls vividly complaining about the fact that there was sometimes only a cold meal for him when he had finished. He made his complaint to the Matron and the Medical Superintendent.

> I said, 'We are working out in this cold weather and in the rain and snow and that's what you think about it — going back to a cold meal.'

When not building walls, Henry worked on the Park farm.

> Oh — cleaning up, feeding hens and that, going round 'streets collecting — used to go round collecting it for 'pigs and that.

Frank, admitted at the same time, remembers having to clean for the staff:

> When I were at Park, first job down at the new lodge — cleaning up for the staff. I used to do all the floors and the bedrooms and that. Every day, upstairs and down — getting it ready for them.

working in the market garden:

> I worked on 'farm over here. We used to plant potatoes and do cabbages and that for the dinners — carrots and all that. Did the fields, them down there where 'school is.

and working in the kitchens:

> I used to do the coppers... like a big tin to boil the tatties and cabbage and all that. We used to fetch it out and scuff it up and that. Used to make sure they were safe and clean.

Admitted a few years later, Horace remembers being set to work on his first day. He was given the job of clearing the recreation hall.

> Sweeping up, polishing the floor — that were on the first day I went.
> I used to go in 'recreation hall, take the mucky laundry up and then go up again and bring the clean laundry. From nine o'clock in the morning 'til five o'clock at night. You have to do your own washing up and you had everyone else's. You had to clean all the floors and polish it. (We were) paid thruppence a week. There used to be a big cig machine outside. I used to put me money in. You got five cigs a penny and matches thrown in.

Horace was a capable young man and was put in charge of a group of four others. During the war, when labour was in short supply, he graduated to a job outside the hospital for which he was paid the comparatively large sum of '£3 in pound notes'.

In the late thirties and early forties the work opportunities for men expanded from cleaning, farming, maintenance and market gardening, to include working in the tailoring department, the joiner's shop, mattress making and the upholsterers. Frank, who seems to have turned his hand to most things, made 'coir mats to wipe your feet on' and 'poultered mattresses' (stuffed them with horse-hair).

Ernest because of his lack of mobility, was set to work in the tailor's shop.

> In the first week I started in the tailor's department of the workshop. I was doing button stitching, stitching buttons on to clothing that came up for repair from the villas. First repairing that was necessary was done by girls who were on the job and anything that was in need of buttons, I used to do that. Mostly on working clothes.
> When the buttons were tested after I'd sewn them on I'd sewn them so tightly that they weren't able to move one way or the other. The man in charge tested them after I had sewn them on.

He remembers some token payment for his work.

> In the first few years of my life here, times were hard. Patients went to work, some on the land, some on the gardens, while the majority of them were on an assortment of different jobs in the workshops. The pay in those days was tuppence weekly. There was an increase, it was one penny and one had to be very careful how one behaved.

Frank worked as a sort of unpaid general factotum for a member of staff who lived in the 'New Lodge' in the hospital grounds.

> I used to work for her. When she used to do washing and all that I used to (work) the wringing machine and she used to peg all the clothes out. She didn't use to pay me and so when 'committee got to know they had to pay me. I used to do a lot of work down there and they didn't use to pay me. I was doing all the work. They didn't pay me when I finished me work — they didn't pay me.
>
> They used to have two daughters and I used to have to shout up and take their meals up. They used to come out (of their bedroom) and take if off me and then I had to go straight downstairs.

Some of the men and some women too had jobs outside the colony. For the women, this work was often domestic service in local houses. For the men, it could involve factory or farm work or some odd-jobbing and gardening for local magnates. A letter addressed to a local baronet in 1944 stated that the charge for labour undertaken by one of the colonists was to be fixed at 7s.6d. per week. Unfortunately, the records do not state whether the colonist or the colony received the money.

The people in this book were the most able residents: because of this, they were set to work in a wide variety of jobs for long hours every day. The villas were cleaned, disabled patients were washed, dressed and cared for, clothes for the whole colony were washed, ironed and repaired, food was cooked, the gardens trimmed and 56 acres of market garden cultivated. Statistical tables dated 1949 show that the market garden contributed well over £1,000 worth of vegetables to the colony's kitchen, in addition to distributing 7 tons of vegetables to other hospitals and marketing a further 4 tons. Grain and oats were also marketed. All this work was labour intensive and carried out with the minimum of technical equipment.

Although their work was crucial to the smooth, efficient and economical running of the colony, this work seems to have been viewed as some sort of atonement to society for the fact that the colonists had been certified as mentally deficient. The workers were unpaid and at the most 'awarded' pocket money which, of course, could be withdrawn for any infringement of the colony's rules. Nevertheless, these people certainly fared better than the less able residents who did not have the same purpose and structure built into their lives and who had little or no opportunity for leaving their villa regularly and for earning even a bar of chocolate or a little extra money. Life for the most disabled and handicapped must have consisted of long empty hours spent waiting for the next meal, for toileting, for bathing and for bedtime. The terms 'boring' and 'just sitting about' are used by physically disabled residents to describe their unoccupied day.

Until the late 1960s, the more severely physically handicapped people were nursed in bed and so had even less stimulation than those who were able to sit in the day-room. A career in bed is now recognised as increasing physical deformities and makes dressing, washing, eating and lifting even more painful and difficult. Some of the more able residents were allocated responsibility for looking after their more handicapped fellows who were universally termed 'babies' or 'low grades'. There was little choice on either side and tired, over-worked residents, like tired, over-worked staff, may sometimes have had little patience with their charges. Certainly, they would have received no training in handling people with such serious physical handicaps.

Work, hard though it was, must have been preferable. Whether paid or unpaid, it did at least offer variety, the status of being acknowledged as 'a high grade' or 'a working girl', the opportunity to meet others, a sense of self-esteem and occasionally praise from members of staff.

7

'On Certain Days, Certain Times, Certain Nights...'

Leisure and Special Events

Colonists had a set time for leisure as for everything else.

> From 5.30 p.m. (after the tea hour) patients should have full advantage of the Recreation Hour so that they may become healthily tired before bedtime. This will have the effect of introducing order and quiet into the dormitories.

It was naturally strictly supervised and controlled.

> During Recreation Hours as far as possible male and female patients should be separated and should play games in groups under the direction of a Nurse Attendant in charge of each group. The games should be organised by the Staff. In inclement weather they should be amused in the recreation rooms with games, toys and other forms of entertainment.

For some, this Recreation Hour represented a real chance to do what they wanted and, for those with talents like Doris, an opportunity to practise and entertain their fellow inmates.

> Used to sit around the fire and read. Do your own knitting and sewing. Some of the girls like me made a concert up, girls in 'villa. (Doris)

Elsie and Margaret greatly appreciated these home-grown entertainments.

> They had big girls and they got a concert up. I used to go and watch them practise. (Elsie)

> I tell you what happened on a Wednesday night, we used to have Highland Fling and dancing. We had record player on villa 10. When there was nothing going off at night we used to have singing and record player. Friday night there weren't anything going off (and) we used to talk to staff. (Margaret)

Grace, who worked so hard all week, used to find that Saturday provided an opportunity for more creative work.

We all used to sit together, friends and do fancy work or knitting or whatever we wanted to do. I did fancy work and anything like that — sewing. If they wanted sewing doing, I used to do it. We never fighted or grumbled for all we hadn't much.

For Margaret, who was physically disabled, the weekend brought little change.

At the weekend we just used to sit out when it was warm. We used to walk round the villas, just your own villa.

The Board of Control Annual Report published in the year The Park was opened recognised the importance of organised leisure in keeping inmates happy, maintaining order and decreasing the numbers of absconders.

Lastly, but certainly not of the least importance, is the organisation of pleasures and amusements for the mentally defective, which should be regarded as one of the ordinary duties of every member of the staff. No institution will be successful in making patients happy and contented to remain unless great attention is paid to this side of colony life.

In the early days of the institution, before there was a recreation hall where the inmates could congregate together, David and Elizabeth and some of the more fortunate were able to attend concerts and dances that were improvised in one of the villas.

The recreation hall weren't up then. They used to have it on 13s and they used to put a screen round for them to get summat for 'concerts. Used to have it on villa 13s, concerts and dances. Used to have a stage there. (David)

Sometimes the old days were good — if you had a concert or somebody had come to play. Sister Morgan, when she were on the villa, she used to make us concerts up and that's the only time I used to like it! And she used to let the lads join with you. (Elizabeth)

Life for the less able must have been monotonous. They had less opportunity for work or occupation and must have sat through many long empty hours every day. If they were unable to entertain themselves, the alternative was the wireless or the gramophone.

We played the radio, listened to the radio. (Joan)

There were no tellies then, only gramophone. Anyway, somebody used to play the gramophone and put it on. All different kinds of music and songs nearly every day and on a night. (Margaret)

Ernest, always self-sufficient, developed his own preferences.

> For my part I used to listen to the radio a lot especially where music was concerned. I was then as I am now, fond of classical music. I used to enjoy music from the theatre and films and orchestral music and piano music.

For those who were children in the early years of The Park, there were, of course, toys. Henry, who was admitted at the age of six, remembers taking some toys and 'drawing books an' that, tracing books' into The Park with him but recalls that these ended up by being 'for somebody else to play with' and that 'somebody took them'. Probably this was the first of a number of lessons about the hazards of communal institutional life.

The need for providing, organising and controlling leisure activities was an important aspect of the smooth functioning of any colony. The planners and providers of care and control deemed necessary for the mentally deficient faced a dilemma. When they were debating the extensions to The Park in the 1930s, they had to decide whether it was or was not morally right and proper to provide facilities for leisure and recreation. The dilemma was a financial one: colonies were designed to place the minimum burden on the community. The economic hardships of the 1930s and the build-up to the Second World War were already taxing the resources of the local community. The provision of leisure activities would add to that burden in what could be viewed as a frivolous and unnecessary way. Much debate surrounded the decision as to whether or not the colony should be provided with a recreation hall. In the end those in favour of the recreation hall had their way.

> In considering the necessity for a recreation hall, it must be remembered that the inmates of a mental deficiency colony are for all practical purposes cut off from the outside world. In these circumstances, the recreation hall becomes an important unit. It can be made to serve such purposes as entertainments, dances, drill and various assemblies, etc. (Annual Report, 1933)

This proposal was not only or even mainly to enhance the quality of life of the inmates but to promote the best interests of the institution.

> Its existence helps very materially not only to provide means to relieve the monotony of colony life, but to foster the community spirit and promote various interests and activities conducive to the health and discipline of the patients.

However, the argument to build a recreation hall was won by compromise. The hall, when completed, should be capable of seating

75 per cent of the inmates, rather than all of them. Presumably some inmates were declared too handicapped to benefit, whilst of the others there would, at any one time, be some confined to their villa because of breaches of institutional discipline. Moreover, the hall was to be of the 'simplest' and presumably therefore the cheapest type of design and construction.

The opening of the recreation hall, 'the centre of the social life of the colony', automatically institutionalised the inmates' free time.

> There were no tellies then, no tellies at all, so the only nights we went out were Saturday nights for concerts, Monday nights for Guides and Thursday nights for pictures. (Margaret)

Getting the inmates to and from the recreation hall was a task that called for order and discipline reminiscent of prisons or army systems.

> They used to have some concert parties coming up to entertain us on a Saturday night in the recreation hall. They had to go from seven-thirty to eight or nine. Patients were lined up outside their villas, those that wanted to go would be checked in number so that they knew, when it was time for them to come back after the show, that the same number that went down were returned. If anyone went missing, which they did occasionally, staff would start a search and if they found the person missing, they would inform the police. When the patient gone missing was finally found they were up before the senior physician.

Once inside the hall, the institution did not slacken its standards.

> All the male patients used to sit on one side of the hall and the female patients on the opposite side. (Ernest)

The recreation hall was licensed for 'Music, Dancing and Cinematograph'. In 1948, the Park's Annual Report proudly announced that it had had twenty-two Saturday concerts as well as weekly film shows. The institution of Thursday films in the recreation hall seems to have been viewed as a mixed blessing. For Frank, Grace and Elizabeth it meant that their trip to the local cinema, 'The Capital', outside The Park was stopped.

> We used to go t' pictures on a Saturday afternoon. Sometimes at that pictures outside The Park. Then they stopped going to that pictures. We'd see 'pictures in 'recreation hall every Thursday. Boys at one side, girls at another. We weren't allowed to sit wi' boys. Weren't supposed to (talk to boys). Dr Black was at 'back. But we used to do. They used to do. (Grace)

Margaret recalls that the pictures lasted from 6.00 to 8.00 p.m. so that inmates were back on their villas in time for the staff shift changes. Instead of having access to films available to the general public, films were now chosen for them and the constant staff surveillance was regarded by all as irksome.

> It used to be 'same when you went to 'pictures — always used to be a staff with you. (The films were) cowboy stuff; nearly always cowboys and indians. I'd have stopped on 'villa if I'd known it were bloody cowboys! You had to have what they said, what they brought. (Elizabeth)

For Frank there was no comparison between the films he had been able to see at the local cinema and those that the recreation hall offered.

> I didn't go much to see the films there. I didn't think they were much good.

A number of people recall that the films were mostly cowboys, 'John Waynes'. None of these recollections seem to have been positive ones; the choice of films either reflected preferences of the staff involved or what was most easily and, again, cheaply available. Ernest summed up the reaction of many.

> I remember there were films on Thursday night and at holiday times. They used to have them twice weekly on Thursday night and Saturday night. A lot of westerns that had been out for a long time and been seen at most of the cinemas outside before coming here. At holiday times we used to see them when they hadn't been out very long, quite recent compared to the other films. I didn't used to go. I used to prefer staying put and listening to music and drama on the radio.

But for those with physical handicaps who had not been allowed out to the local cinema or church, the recreation hall did increase their opportunities to experience something different. George appreciated the fact that there were 'plenty of shows', as did Margaret and Joan.

Besides concerts and films, the recreation hall was used for the institution's fancy dress dance.

> We used to have fancy dress, but we used to get dressed up funny. You know like them mask things for your face. We'd make something on the villa like for fancy dress. It were really nice in the olden days. (Margaret)

For hard-working and creative Grace, the fancy dress party offered an opportunity to show off her talents.

Leisure and Special Events 85

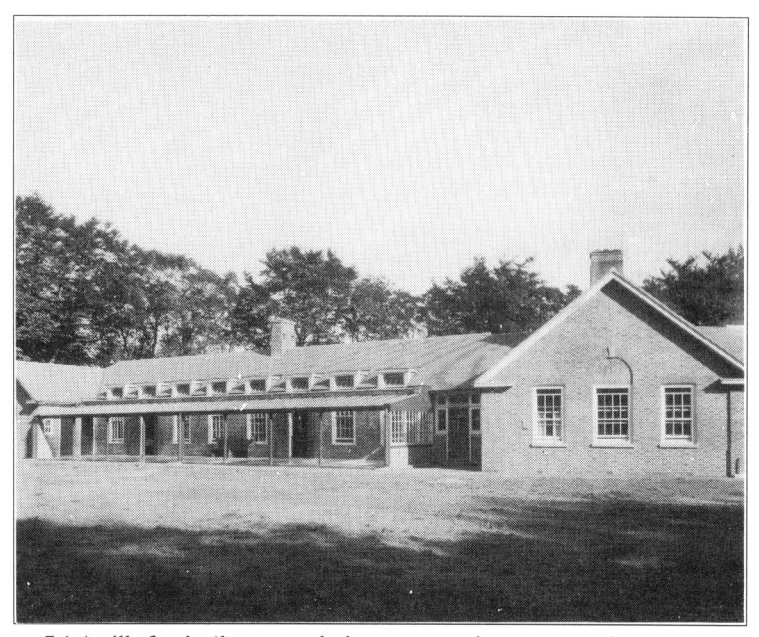

7.1 A villa for the 'lowest grades' to accommodate twenty males and twenty females. Official opening, 1932.

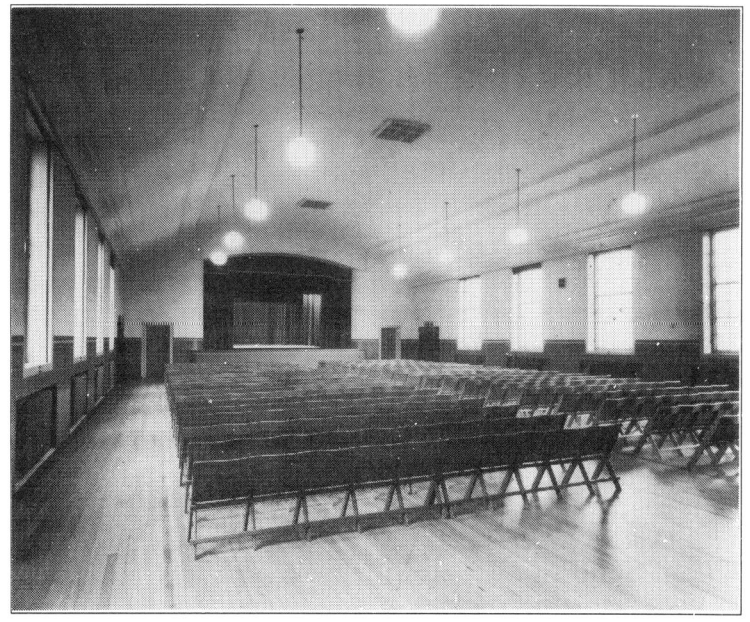

7.2 'The Recreation Hall provides seating for six-hundred persons and is intended to form the centre of the social life of the colony.' Official opening, 1941.

I used to dress up for fancy dress. I won first prize me. I got dressed up as all sorts. I once was an old tinker with a frying-pan at back of me back and torn trousers and I got first prize.

In dancing particularly, strict regard was paid to the way that the male and female colonists behaved with one another.

The girls used to dance with the girls and the boys used to dance with the boys. Some people might have danced with a boy. I think staff were looking to see, keeping their eye on them to see if they were up to mischief. (Margaret)

They used to give us Christmas dances and do's... That were all right but you couldn't mix. Lads had to have it altogether and girls on their own. (Elizabeth)

As standards changed in more recent times, men were sometimes allowed to ask a woman to dance but they had to do so properly and in accordance with the rules of etiquette.

We used to go dancing. Females at that end and males at this end. Used to go and say, 'Can I have the honour of this dance, please?' (Henry)

The local authority planners in their efforts not to appear to be providing unnecessarily luxurious facilities for the inmates also designed the recreation hall to be used for religious services. Reading through reports of the time this seems to have been a hotly debated issue: a number of those involved argued for a separate, properly dedicated church. Although the Planning Committee accepted that 'many defectives are open to spiritual appeal and derive great benefit from religious services', they did not feel that this deserved to be recognised through the building of a chapel, and concluded that:

However, while we cannot recommend the provision of a separate chapel as an essential requirement, we gladly repeat a suggestion made to us that the gift of a colony chapel by private benefaction or through local philanthropy would be a gracious and sympathetic act.

Unfortunately, no-one ever made such a gift to The Park and religious services were held in the recreation hall until its closure in 1987. Certainly the Committee were correct in the case of one resident: Ernest did derive great benefit from religious services and, with the help of a sympathetic member of staff, held religious services in his own villa.

The Friday service meetings that I used to hold were between 5.30 and 7.30 p.m. Muriel and I took it in turns, reading lessons and announcing the hymns. I was started off by one of the nursing staff here because he was interested in that kind of thing. I was interested in anything to do with church business and the staff knew that I was interested. In those meetings there were always the patients on the villa that I was on. There were also some other friends that I had from other villas.

When the time came and Mr Thomas went off the villa and went to another villa, then things were at a standstill until Mr Grant came and I spoke to him and they were restarted again.

Initiatives of this kind were absolutely dependent on the goodwill of staff and their willingness to circumvent the tyranny of routine. These services ceased when Ernest's health deteriorated and he, like others, was forced to be at the mercy of that same routine: the need to have him washed, dressed and ready for bed before the night staff are on duty.

Because the routine has changed with me and the staff's dealings with me. After tea and they've had their own break, I'm brought down here for getting undressed and toileting to change into my nightclothes and then (I) spend the evening watching television until the night staff come on duty.

If the planners had felt that building a chapel was a luxury that was not really necessary, this view was certainly not shared by Doris, Frank or Elizabeth who were acutely aware that something important to them had been taken away and replaced by second best.

Go to that recreation hall. We didn't go down to the village church, the outside church. Sunday afternoon, I used to go for a bit. I didn't always go 'cos I didn't like... I said, this isn't church. That isn't a church, it's only a... (Doris)

The advent of church in the recreation hall was a real curtailment of their very limited contact with the outside world. First trips to the local cinema became unnecessary and now worshipping in a local church was prevented.

Staff used to be with you — wouldn't let you go outside to church. That all got stopped. That's why they made that recreation hall — made it into a church for Sundays. They made it into a picture house and it used to be 'same when you went to 'pictures, always used to be a staff with you. (Elizabeth)

Other regular features of institutional life at The Park were meetings of the colony's own Girl Guides and Trefoil Guild and the Boy Scout Group and Rovers. The Scouts and Guides did provide inmates with formal links to the outside world. Both were inspected by District Commissioners and took part in activities with other groups outside the colony. The Guides took part in parades and garden parties, whilst the Scouts seem to have been more adventurous, taking part in meetings outside the colony and, on at least one occasion, acting as hosts to the District Rovers at a weekend camp. Both Scouts and Guides wore uniforms and both seem to have conducted their business in ways that were very similar to other Scout and Guide groups in the community. There was one important difference, however — The Park's Scouts and Guides were men and women, not boys and girls.

> We used to have Guides in the patients' school on a Monday night 6.30 till 7.30. We used to wear them uniforms, black skirts and blue ties. Guides laws, promise and me honour — things like that. (Margaret)

For Guides, the activities were mainly of a leisure and recreational variety and were directly influenced by 'the enthusiasm and skill at handicraft hobbies' of the leader (Annual Report, 1949).

On the other hand, for men, the Scouts were seen as 'an active feature of colony training'. From available pictures and the memories of the Scouts in the colony, the two main activities were the Scout band and gymnastics. Gymnastic displays by the Scouts were one of the principle features of sports days and The Park's archives contain a great many pictures of these displays. They show muscular men, in baggy shorts, balanced one on top of the other in various set pieces.

The Scout band was held in considerable esteem.

> We had one of the best bands going. (Henry)

This band was a bugle band which seems to have become the institution's pride and joy. One of the colony's Annual Reports states that 'their skill compared favourably with similar bands in the local Scouts.' This bugle band gave the colonists not only something to be proud of, but a legitimate place in the local community. One man remembers the band taking part in a 'big parade in Town Hall'. The bugle band took part in regular Sunday afternoon parades.

> On a Sunday Boy Scouts used to come up, every Sunday afternoon. I can't remember if they were from outside or from here but they used to come up every Sunday you know. Play drums and them flags, used to clap you know. (Margaret)

For Margaret, it emphasised the difference between being a Scout and only being a Guide.

> On a Sunday afternoon we used to have Scouts parade, flags and drums. They played drums and waved them flags. We only used to clap.

It was also in demand for dances in the newly erected recreation hall.

> Used to have dancing. They all come up to you to dance wi' you. Just the Scouts to play. (Horace)

Probably the most important event in the colony's life was the opening of the extensions in 1941 by the Princess Royal. This was the opportunity for the Scouts and Guides to be on parade, as Horace remembers:

> Scouts were there when Princess Royal was opening it. Henry used to be in 'Scouts. There used to be a Scout parade. Used to march all round the villas and back to the Scout huts. (Horace)

Press pictures of the time show the Scouts and Guides in immaculate uniforms standing to attention whilst they were being inspected by the Princess Royal.

Listening to the recorded memories and looking through Annual Reports, a strong impression is gained that leisure for women colonists was much less organised and varied and at the same time much more insular and controlled. For women, leisure time was spent in useful handicrafts or games such as cards, in occasional well-chaperoned dances or, of course, the film shows. At weekends, apart from church, they seem to have 'stopped on villa'. The 1948 Annual Report states that some of the younger women played netball and took part in dancing and eurhythmic classes which were 'organised and instructed by the matron and the head teacher'. None of the women could remember these activities and it seems likely that they were restricted to young women in their late teens. This same report listed the favourite indoor amusements as needlecraft, cards, music and dancing.

For men, however, activities provided a sanctioned outlet for physical energy, aggression and sexual drive. For them leisure therefore involved opportunities for physical exercise and competition. The 1948 report listed the recreation and play activities for males as follows:

> During the appropriate seasons cricket and football matches were arranged and parties of patients visited local matches. Inter-villa competitions were held and billiards, cards, ring-boards and dominoes were popular indoor amusements.

Physical activity offered an outlet for pent-up frustration and a chance to be successful. This difference between opportunities for men and women is clearly seen in the arrangements made for physical exercise: for men it was cricket and football, 'Fridays outside', and a chance to play against local teams, but for women it was the supervised walk. Grace, who looked after her niece, a resident on one of the other villas, managed to escape the tedium of those walks.

> On a Sunday we used to have to go out in all weathers, round the block while four o'clock. All round 'walls, where 'walls are. I didn't, I used to go to villa 2 and look after Doreen. We used to go out at night-time after tea when they got 'doors open. (Grace)

One of the special events of the year was the annual sports day: the sports being adapted for the less able-bodied residents.

> Used to have different sports. There were races for those who could run and we also included another one for the slow walkers. In their case it were the slow walkers who were different from the ones able to do the running. First one was a prize winner and in the slow walkers it was the last one. I remember one time I won one of the prizes for that. It was a case of people going as slow as they could rather than running for those that were able to run. (Ernest)

This was an important event with prizes and a shield to be won. For some, staff as well as colonists, it was a splendid opportunity to vent their feelings.

> When you had sports day used to have egg and spoon race. Used to go round villas and pass this thing to other people and when you come back had to pass this stick to 'next person. And the last that come in used to get prizes, sweets and a shield. Used to have blind boxing when someone had a go at Dr Black's face!
> After sports were finished, down to 'recreation hall for a dance. It were a band that come. (Horace)

The other great institutional event was Christmas. This was the celebration that stimulated some of the happiest memories recounted. The first signs of Christmas in the colony were seen at school.

> You had to start drawing pictures of Santa Claus and reindeer and everything like that. (Henry)

The more able residents were allowed to go down to town with staff.

> Well, they used to take us out at Christmas for Christmas Day shopping. I

used to go down on 'tram'. (Frank)

Carol singing, parties, dances and decorations were all part of Christmas for these men and women. Horace and Henry remember going round the villas, including ones where the most disabled people lived, and wishing them a 'Merry Christmas' and singing. The men, in particular, recall being allowed to go 'round the villas to the girls' side'. Christmas dances were held in the recreation hall where there was 'a bloke who dressed up as Santa'. Until the early 1980s, there was a Christmas show every year. For Tom, this increased the choices he was able to make.

> Used to be a show every Christmas, dancing and parties (or) just stopped in 'villas.

Parties on the villas depended upon staff's preferences.

> Sometimes we had parties depending on who happened to be on duty. If there was somebody who was fond of arranging anything like that then they used to do so. Food was very different from the ordinary food. (Ernest)

Not everyone remembers Christmas as something special: for Violet it was just another day.

> Just about the same, I think. Nobody came. (Violet)

Christmas Day itself was one of the few days of rest for the colonists, who recalled the atmosphere of mutual goodwill.

> We didn't go to work that day, Christmas Day, Boxing Day and New Year's Day. (Henry)

> Christmas Day staff said, 'You've done well, you've worked hard.' (Horace)

For the younger residents, like Joan and Margaret, the excitement was contagious.

> They used to say, 'Hurry up. Let's get breakfast over with then you can see your presents.'

Presents were for opening after breakfast only. (Margaret)

> Have breakfast and all the presents were out. I used to like opening mine. You could get all sorts of presents. A dolly (was favourite) when I was a little girl. (Joan)

A number of people recognised that their presents were provided for them and that they had little choice: however, this does not seem to have soured their enthusiasm for Christmas.

> We couldn't go out and buy presents 'cos we had no money but they used to, you know the Government, they used to send presents. Like once they sent me a bed-jacket and like bed-socks. One time they sent chocolate, but you didn't get much, like you do now, you can go and buy your own. (Henry)

> I got quite a few (presents); some books, some crayons, pair of socks, tie, some got pullovers. The National Insurance people were only ones that sent them and to other places. Well they do that National Insurance, don't they. I'm glad they do. (Horace)

> It weren't a case of choosing (presents), you had to be content with whatever you received which I was happy about. I used to always receive something that was of some use to me. I was happy about that. (Ernest)

Villas were sometimes elaborately decorated for Christmas and Christmas dinner was a special meal, 'A nice dinner', although for Henry it was marred by the lack of alcohol.

> Couldn't go out for a drink then. Used to drink orange juice.

Writing in 1974, Ernest recalls a vivid Christmas dream:

> When some people dream it is surprising how real and life-like our dreams can be. So much so that we expect to wake up in the morning to find them come true and as true as they appeared. I remember experiencing something like this myself some years ago. (I cannot remember exactly how long ago.) I was in the General Hospital at the time, recovering from diphtheria. It was Christmas Eve and as I slept I dreamed that on Christmas morning when I received my presents, amongst them was a box of those dominoes with the coloured spots and on receiving them and having looked through the rest of my presents, I had put the dominoes under my pillow. The first thing I did on awakening on Christmas morning was to look under my pillow only to be disappointed to find that the box of dominoes was not there. (From *My life at The Park*, 1974)

Judging from the pictures of Christmas cakes for each of the villas, the skills of the colony's cooks were considerable: cakes for each villa were elaborately decorated and distinctly different. One of the school teachers, who worked at the colony just after the war, remembers these cakes and their icing which was so hard that Dr Black had difficulty in cutting it.

Leisure and Special Events 93

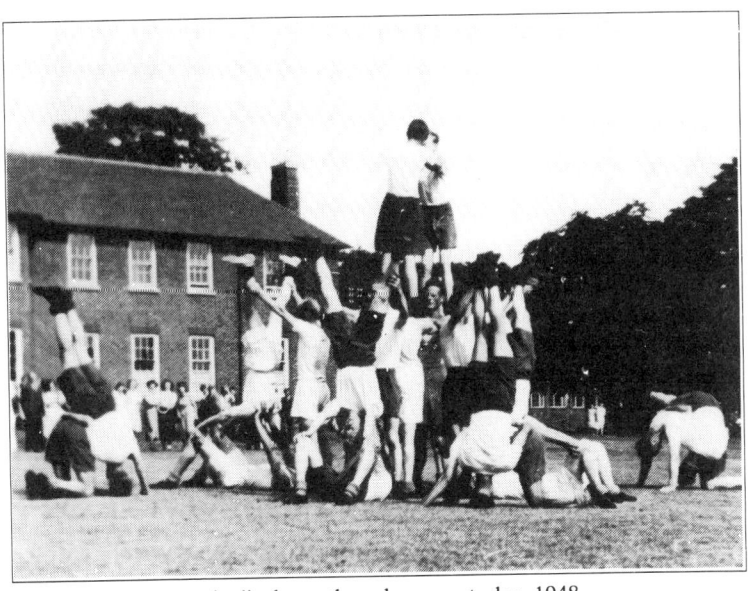

7.3 Scout gymnastic display at the colony sports day, 1948.

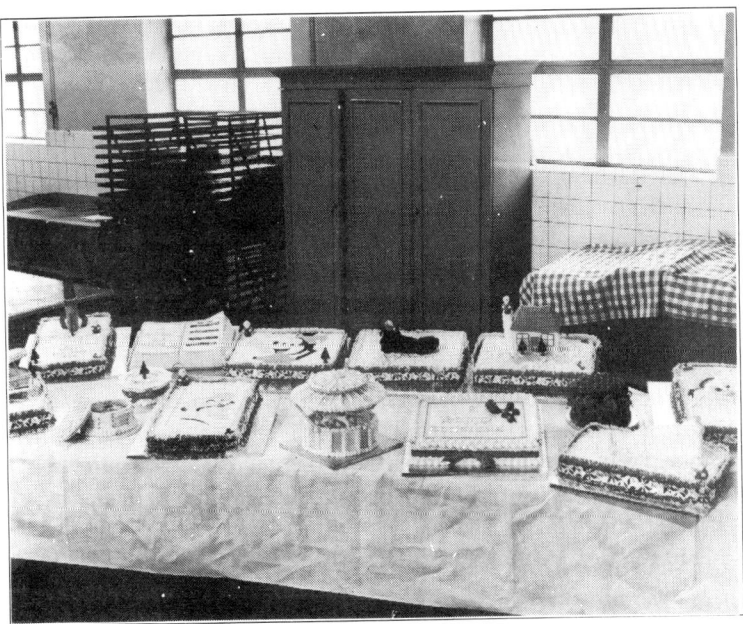

7.4 Colony Christmas cakes, circa 1950.

Christmas at the colony was the result of the successful combination of institutional resources which overcame, for the Christmas period at least, the inbuilt disadvantages of lack of money and little freedom of choice. Personal celebrations such as birthdays, however, are remembered by very few people. Two men remember being given a birthday party which was all right, one man adding that he 'didn't think about birthdays at all.' For children in the colony, birthdays may have received more recognition.

> They used to give us (a party) on us birthday — give us a do. I won't say they didn't give us them things like that 'cos they did. (Grace)

Henry remembers that when he was seven years old,

> They used to buy me some little pairs of socks, a jersey or some mittens or a small pair of boots.

But when he was an adult, he didn't even receive clothing, in fact nothing special distinguished the day.

> You didn't do owt. I didn't bother. (Henry)

The official view of leisure was not that it was to be enjoyed for its own sake, but that it was a useful safety-valve providing legitimate outlets for frustration, aggression and other unacceptable feelings. It was very strictly controlled. Although the recreation hall may have offered a chance to join in social activities for some of the less able people, for the more able it reduced their freedom of movement. For them the institution became total: regular contact with the outside at church or at the cinema ceased. The institution could now play together as well as work together.

If leisure and recreation activities appear to have been directed primarily at the most able residents, then holidays and day-trips in the early years of the institution were almost exclusively reserved for the able-bodied. Their work was essential to the smooth running of the institution: the occasional day-trip or holiday may have been simply another way of helping them to be more content with their lot. One charge nurse, in his own reminiscences, stated that the patients were selected for holidays and outings by the Chief Male Nurse and the Medical Superintendent, no doubt on the recommendation of the nursing staff. Since such events were privileges, not rights, there was probably plenty of scope for favouritism.

The 1930 Annual Report mentions a day-trip into the country for women whilst the men had a holiday at the seaside. In fact, in terms of holidays, yet again men seemed to fare better than women. In 1934, 'high-grade' men from the colony joined other men who lived at home but attended the local Occupation Centre for a holiday at a YMCA camp. In 1935, a holiday for sixty men is mentioned in the Annual Report, and further references to holidays for men are made in 1937. Margaret recalls the day-trips and the absence of holidays:

> They used to go on day-trips you know . . . we didn't go a long way because it was just day-trips. You know like we do now, go on holiday, we never used to go on holiday like we do now.
>
> They used to take us out for the day. I used to play in the sand. They used to sit me down in the sand. (Margaret)

In 1938, fifty men had a holiday. However, 1938 represents something of a landmark for the women of the colony. In order to relieve the overcrowding on the villas, the Committee leased a holiday home in the Lake District which served the dual purpose of relieving overcrowding on the villas and enabling some villas to move lock, stock and barrel for a nice safe holiday all together.

> Everybody (on the villa), nurses and staff. It were a nice place. We used to go there for a fortnight. It were a nice, big house. (Grace)

Ninety-six people, including sixteen women, spent twelve weeks at this holiday home in the summer of 1938. In the winter, a similar number, but this time all men, were transferred there for a few months to relieve pressure on the villas, whilst the new extensions were being completed. In 1940, this treat stopped because of staffing difficulties which were exacerbated by the war. Not surprisingly, little mention is made of holidays or day-trips during the war years: the only one noted in reports was an outing to the grounds of a house that was formerly one of the colony's annexes. However, Ernest, who was admitted just after the war, remembers holidays clearly and confirms the impression that it was the most able who benefited.

> The patients who could do certain things that the others couldn't, reading, writing, spelling, doing numbers, things like that. (It was) the ones that could do them that were included on the holidays. There were a number of people in wheelchairs taken. I was one of the ones who went. At that time I was able to walk. (Ernest)

For school trips, too, the headmistress selected the most able pupils.

Those who were left behind had to move house as well. In the interests of economy, the villa had to be closed whilst the others were away. Those who did not go on holiday were referred to by Ernest as,

> The not so sensible ones. I thought it should be possible for them to be included. I didn't see no reason why they should be left out. Some of them made their feelings known by speaking out about it — only amongst themselves, of course.
>
> If all the patients on the villa where I was were taken, the ones that didn't go were mixed in amongst the patients on another villa until they came back. So the villa was locked. Some of them were a bit down and out. The others mixed in with the ones that had been left behind, spoke in a friendly way to them and they took part in any form of enjoyment that took place on the villa they'd been left on. Some of them may have been upset but when they got into conversation and friendships with others that were left behind, they didn't let their feelings known so much.

After the war, more people can remember going away for a holiday. In 1949, eighty-eight patients went on a camp for a week but this was 'marred by inclement weather'. Although large numbers of colonists all went together and stayed together, so that it was, in effect, the institution on holiday, it nevertheless offered unprecedented freedom from staff surveillance for a lucky few.

> Used to go Blackpool for a week's holiday and go out on your own with your spending money. And you had to go out on your own and be back just in time for meals. Well after the war that was. (Horace)

Although there were no holidays and few day-trips during the war, this event was, for The Park, very special indeed. The war meant soldiers. Like many institutions at the time, part of the site was commandeered to provide hospital facilities for the wounded; not only British wounded soldiers, but German prisoners of war as well. Although there must have been well over 300 British and German soldiers on site, no mention is made of their presence in the reports of the time, presumably for security reasons. Accommodating soldiers meant creating room by doubling up on some of the villas. All the new villas which had been opened by the Princess Royal seemed to have been occupied by soldiers for the duration of the war.

> I were here when air-raid were on, soldiers and Germans and all 'lot. They (the new villas) were only built for the soldiers. There was villa 9 full of soldiers. They weren't allowed to talk to us through 'day. I don't know whether they were Germans or not; there were some Germans here. What's

villa 4 now used to be full of soldiers. (Elizabeth)

Some of our soldiers came in on villa 17. When they built the villas, they went in did 'soldiers. Ambulance used to keep bringing 'em up when they got lamed and all that. They put so many on villa 15 and then they put so many in 14 when it got up. And when villa 9 were put up, then 'Germans went in. Then on villa 9, we hadn't to go over 'cos they were Germans. (David)

Villa 4 was for old ladies before they (the soldiers) took it over. (Frank)

Official history does not record just how many people were moved or where they all went. Some people can recall some of the movements.

They moved a lot out for them to go in, some on the villas. (Doris)

During the war 13s' patients got moved off because 13s used to be a hospital. (Tom)

Since the colony had been designed for the sexes to be strictly segregated, it was very easy for the British and German soldiers to be kept separate.

Soldiers, some from Germany and our British soldiers. Germans stayed on where the female side is, villa 9, that's all. (Horace)

For the authorities, putting German prisoners of war on the female side and unguarded British soldiers on the male side was no doubt intended to prevent female residents fraternising with the soldiers.

All them soldiers, they were all in villa 4 and villa 3 and villa 8. They were all in and me father used to come once a month. We couldn't talk to them. And I weren't to go over there where they were. They used to sit out, outside. (Doris)

However, here as anywhere else, rules were made to be broken and Grace recalls clandestine encounters with British soldiers.

Soldiers, they were on 'male side. Girls used to like 'em. We used to get lovely boxes of chocolates. We used to go upstairs to eat 'em. They treat us. A soldier would come and say, 'Don't say nowt', 'No, I won't say nowt.' They had to be in for a certain time you see. They were nice. (Grace)

Frank and Joe found the soldiers very friendly.

They put some soldiers up there on 'villas and German people an' all. They were separate. I used to talk with one and he used to give me cigs he did — the Camel ones, they weren't half strong. (Joe)

Despite the fact that the soldiers' presence meant overcrowding and having the enemy in their midst, there is little feeling of rancour or resentment from any of the participants. The soldiers seem to have brought variety, interest, opportunities and supplies.

They were all right, they'd give you a few cigarettes. (Frank)

We didn't go that short of stuff while 'war were on, you know for villas and that.

The soldiers provided yet more work for the able-bodied inmates. It was estimated that during the war some 60 per cent of the colonists were employed in colony work in one way or another.

When 'war were on we looked after 'soldiers. (Grace)

I used to wash up on a night if they wanted any help. (Frank)

I was still working, helping them out. Helping the wounded, helping them out. There were some in wheelchairs, wheeling them round. (Horace)

The war, of course, meant air-raids and gas masks. There was at least one air-raid shelter.

They used to have one of those doings (siren) that went off, used to have to go down in a trench. That were where villa 9s were. When it went, we had to all get out of bed and we had to put us dressing-gowns on and lay flat on us tummy and then after it we had to get up. (David)

When there was an air-raid on, used to use fire doors and rush past, right near 'school and have to go inside the air-raid shelter. You had to switch all the lights off and had black-out curtains as well. We had blinds, black blinds. Had to pull them down so they wouldn't see us. (Henry)

Joe was involved in digging out a place for the shelter.

They had an air-raid shelter outside. I made it, I did and put some lights in it. So when 'sirens went we all went in that air-raid shelter. (Joe)

Conditions in the shelter were cramped and damp.

The air-raid shelter was at 'back of villa 9. Used to run down there. It were awful, water in and that. (Tom)

The air-raids provided opportunities for the more adventurous and desperate inmates: the chance of making a run for it in the confusion was one that some people couldn't resist.

> I remember running out t' air-raid shelter. I remember a few of them running off in there. And when we were at 'shelter somebody'd come up and say 'Have you seen so-and-so? Do you know where she is?' I says, 'Don't ask me, I don't know where she is. I'm not her boss, she can go where she likes.' 'Cos she ran away with somebody. (Elizabeth)

Only the able-bodied could use the air-raid shelter, others had to remain on the villa.

> We had to come in 'day-room, brought blankets down and laid on blankets in the day-room. And then we went back upstairs. We didn't go out at all, outside. (Doris)

Air-raids and short rations had their effect on catering arrangements.

> Food were awful them days. Sometimes we used to drink cold water instead of tea. They didn't use to make it. We had to get used to drinking cold water and dry bread. (Henry)

At the end of the war, the colony was intact and no damage had been done. The colony was now able to return to its original purpose as soldiers left.

> I came on 24 March 1945, three months after I came that's when it ended. Some soldiers who had been injured were on some of the villas. On the same side as villa 13 to 17, but not so many of them as I would have expected to see. (Ernest)

Villas were handed back but changes had to be made before colonists could occupy them again.

> Villa 4 — that villa's altered a lot. They left did soldiers that'd finished and they made it all different again for 'patients, for us. (Elizabeth)

8

'There Was Some Just Hiding Their Feelings'

Social and Sexual Relations

Despite the official guidance that officers should build up trust through the development of a good relationship with parents and their son/daughter, the certification process itself took little account of the feelings of the children and adults who were subjected to it. People labelled mentally defective were dealt with under the Mental Deficiency Act 1913 and were disposed of as was most economically convenient. Since the chief purpose of the Act and the colonies that spawned from it was to prevent the mentally deficient 'repeating their type', relationships were strictly institutionalised and controlled.

Moving abruptly from the security of family life to a large impersonal institution must have struck terror into old and young alike. The colony's first concern was to ensure that the inmates became part of the colony as quickly as possible. One of the most important ways of achieving this was to sever the new inmate from family and friends until he or she had 'settled in'.

Grace, who was admitted when she was seventeen years old, remembers this vividly.

> You'd got to get settled in before they'd let you have any visitors. You'd got to get settled in first for a fortnight. I think it did good, as you'd realise that ... if they let you have visitors, you might just run out with them. That's what they thought. I used to cry when me mother went home.

Joan's parents were anxious about the welfare of their daughter. She was only eight years old when she was admitted and both her mother and her father made verbal and written requests to visit her. Her father was admonished in a letter from the Medical Superintendent that 'it is necessary to adhere strictly to the regular visiting times' and further informed that he would have to wait until the end of the month.

After this settling-in period and when the inmate could have no doubt that this was where she was going to stay, contact with relatives was resumed, but entirely on the colony's terms: two hours once a month.

> They (visitors) were sat with you all the time at the table. Two o'clock when they opened it up, they had to stay outside — queue up. They weren't allowed in. They had to wait till the door was opened. Then they used to go in (the dining-room) for visitors. Sat there till four, once a month. Then they changed it so that people could come at night. (Elizabeth)

Far from it being a right to see one's parents and relatives, it was a special privilege that could be bestowed on those who had kept to the rules, or withdrawn from those who infringed them. Not surprisingly, visiting days were eagerly awaited and the whole colony was on its best behaviour.

> We didn't half look forward to visiting day. (Grace)

> Well, we used to get up on Saturday morning early and used to get dressed up nice, you know, in case we got visitors. (Margaret)

> We all wore us own clothes, all nice new clothes, if anybody came to see us. (Joan)

Relatives, then as now, were an important source, not only of emotional support, but also of small comforts and luxuries not available in the colony.

> When your parents brought you stuff, it were all right. Me mother used to bring me all sorts, and me brothers and sisters. (Grace)

Grace was lucky enough to have regular visits from her parents, who patently cared about her very much.

> Mother visited every month, never missed. She was little and small, but she never missed me: she'd buy me frocks, buy me fruit.

For others, these visiting times were not quite such happy occasions. Relatives and inmates had a whole month in which to build up expectations. Small wonder, then, if visits often fell far short in providing mutual comfort. Relatives coming to visit must have experienced some of the same anxiety, uncertainty and fear that is so vividly recalled by many of the residents in the first few weeks of their entering the colony. Some relatives may also have brought with them ambivalent feelings of guilt and blame for their offspring's incarceration and condition.

Tensions were further increased by the fact that visitors were received in the main day-room, where the lack of privacy made the discussion of personal matters tense and difficult. Everything could be overheard by other relatives, staff and residents. With only this one opportunity a month, it is small wonder that family grievances reached explosion point by the time visiting came round again. Many people can remember visiting being punctuated by rows. Henry can remember when he was a child, visitors coming to his villa, who argued with each other.

> They fall out. I'm not having owt to do with this arguing.

Margaret experienced an unhappy occasion when her parents visited.

> Yes, on an afternoon. But while me Mum and Dad didn't live together, I knew what was going on. I couldn't talk or anything... because me Mum and Dad were having a row. When they came to see me they got chucked out and it upset me because I knew what was going on.
> They were rowing about something and they got sent out. I was crying, you know, in me own way — tears.
> I couldn't talk you know, but I knew all that was going on because they once had a row and now that's why I think they still don't live together.

Many people did not have visitors. Visiting their sons/daughters in the colony may have proved just too daunting for some parents. Some of those who were not visited affected not to care.

> I didn't bother, no, I kept to myself — kept out of mischief. I didn't bother with them. (Joe)

Although Sally did have some visitors, she felt rejected by her family:

> Me brother's first wife, she come a few times. It were only her and me brother what come, never saw anybody else. Me oldest brother, I've never seen him and I've never seen me sister. I felt as if I weren't wanted.

Others had 'no-one to care' for them. Many people were, however, upset by not having visitors. Residents and visitors alike seem to have been sensitive to this.

> There were some just hiding their feelings, but there are others that are able to spend the time in the company of the more fortunate ones, who do have visitors. The visitors are equally ready and prepared to welcome them, make them feel part of the family. (Ernest)

> Some of them had no-one to see them. They hadn't their parents, that's why.

Me mother used to give 'em some of mine. She used to bring them in to sit with us. It was sad for them. (Grace)

For Joan and Henry, a friend's visitors became their visitors as well, and helped to strengthen the bonds between them.

I didn't used to have any — you know Brenda's Aunty Carrie and Uncle George, I knew them since I were on villa 10. (Joan)

I had me mother to come and see us, and Henry used to come down and talk to 'em. We used to sit and talk and make 'em a cup of tea. They'd bring me and him some cigs. (Horace)

Visits from parents and relatives were a reminder of the outside world, an important point of contact with their old life and with their own identity. In controlling contact with parents and relatives, the colony operated, as ever, a hierarchical system of rewards, whose ultimate aim was to ensure maximum work from the able-bodied inmates. People who were unfortunate enough to be more severely handicapped physically or mentally had very little chance of increasing their contact with people outside. A maximum of one visit per month was the most that could be hoped for, provided they remained physically well and kept within the rules. For those who were more able, there was the possibility of earning the much prized visit or holiday at home on parole.

When they found out I was higher grade, then you got a lot more privileges to what the others did. You could do more, you see. (Grace)

Visits home to relatives and unescorted visits outside were felt to encourage habits of 'regular work and good conduct'. 'The hope of securing these privileges stimulates good conduct in the more intelligent and stable patients.' (Yearly Report 1949)

Grace remembers her joy when she was recognised by the institution as 'a high grade' and was granted parole.

When that parole come out, about going out shopping outside. I got it first. Went shopping in the High Street. Then I started going home for me holidays on me own for the weekend. I used to go from Saturday till Sunday and come back on me own. It were lovely. I never though I would, but I did get it. I used to come back as good as gold. I think that's why I got on really. I didn't get funny ideas. Sometimes me sister come wi' me just for company but I was as good as gold.

I couldn't believe it when I were going home on me own. When I were getting on the bus, that's when I couldn't believe it. I couldn't sleep that night, I couldn't believe it!

One surprising memory recounted by three or four residents was that, when they went on parole, they had to have their parole card stamped at the Lodge and had to pay a sum of money ('tuppence'), both when leaving the institution and when returning to it. If this is so, then it means that these people had to work physically very hard to earn their parole and then had to pay for it out of their own pockets as well.

Privileges such as parole did not only depend on the institution's goodwill, but also upon having relatives who were willing to petition the institution for permission to have their patients at home on a visit and were prepared to brave the stigma of the institution by collecting them. Grace's mother was not prepared to tolerate the stigma of institutional clothing and resorted to helping her change her clothes in the churchyard:

My mother used to change mine in 'graveyard.

If patients had caring relatives who accepted their institutional background, then visits home meant new freedoms.

I know I asked him (doctor) once. He says, 'You can't go home.' I says, 'Can I go home on my own?' He says, 'Every patient has to have parents come for them.' They had to come for us when we were on us leave. Not only me, but everybody. We couldn't even go home on us own.

We had to have somebody with us and somebody had to fetch us for our holidays and take us back.

My sister says, 'You can't come home on your own and can't go anywhere on your own, (but) you can do it while you're here. Go where you like while you're on your holidays. I don't wanna go out with you when you do your shopping. You can go on your own, you're old enough. You're not there now!' (Elizabeth)

For Elizabeth, although granted the privilege by the institution, visits home were impossible.

They (my family) wouldn't get me home. They wouldn't have me in for 'holidays. If it hadn't been for her (my sister) at Scotland, I don't know where I'd be now.

For Sally, home visits also meant fresh opportunities for

disagreements, misunderstandings and recriminations.

> When I went to see me brother once and he got mad with me just 'cos I were talking about the olden days. He said, 'What you talking about 'old days for? Can't you talk about summat else?!' He started off a row, 'If you'd 've got up for the mill you'd never been there.' I said I've done me punishment for that and he got so mad he walked out.
> He took it out on his wife 'cos she was sticking up for me. Then when he came back he apologised and said, 'I'm sorry for what I said.' He said, 'You had me trailing up there to see you.' I said, 'I didn't ask you. It wouldn't 've mattered to me if you hadn't come.'

Contact with families and relatives was important to most people. The size of the institution, its location at the northern edge of a large population and its inflexibility to individual needs, all contrived to make contact with relatives difficult and unsatisfactory. Where relationships between residents and their relatives were poor, the system did not help to improve them.

The institution paid scant attention to the feelings of Elizabeth, when her child was taken from her. Indeed, her natural emotional reactions to this even were judged simply as evidence of 'childishness' and hence of mental defect. Her pregnancy and the subsequent birth of her child severed relationships with her parents and with the sister who looked after Elizabeth's child. These events hurt Elizabeth deeply and have left permanent scars.

> They (other people's relatives) haven't been as cruel as what mine have.

However, she did have one person in the family who cared about her, understood her feelings and protected her interests.

> I'm thankful I've got another sister. She's the one that stuck by me all the way through. Because when they (parents) did die, they left everything to the three of them; her in Scotland, her in England, her what died. He (father) left them some money. Her in Scotland said, 'What about Elizabeth? She's a right to have half of it as for us.' She said, 'She's his daughter — our sister as well.' She says, 'Her that died, she's nothing to do with it, she's not here.' She says, 'I'm going to stick up for her. She's gonna have half of it, what there is.' If it hadn't been for her I wouldn't of had none of that money. And I've still got a bit of it now in 'bank outside.

If institutional rules made it difficult to maintain relationships with relatives, institutional practices seemed to be designed to prevent residents from forming relationships with each other.

As you got older, you got moved. (Grace)

Being moved about the institution, especially for the more able residents, was a fact of life. Tom, now happily living in a flat with George, recalls.

> They said they're getting someone else in your place. To be honest I've been on every villa in the hospital except on the female side. I used to have a lot (of friends). Each villa I've gone to I found friends just like that (snaps fingers).
> (So what about leaving them when you moved villas?)
> That's stupid! That's what used to happen. Didn't like it. I used to go visiting on 'villas every night when I can get out. I used to sneak out. Had to let staff know in case owt happened.

Being physically handicapped did have one advantage: since ground floor accommodation was scarce, people who needed wheelchairs were not often moved. Joan, Ernest and Margaret are physically handicapped and have lived together for years. They are now an established group who offer mutual help and support. Margaret interprets for Joan, whose speech is very difficult to understand because of the spasticity of her muscles. She also interprets for another member of the group, Brenda:

> Yes, Brenda and me have always been friends together 'cos we were on villa 10 together. That's why I know her Aunty Carrie and Uncle George.

> I help Brenda. Sometimes people can't understand what she says and I help her.

George, who is also physically handicapped, and his flatmate Tom became friends whilst living in the institution and they wanted to move out into the community together. Their friendship has grown and developed since the move. However, the experiences of George and Tom, and Margaret and her friends, are the exception rather than the rule. Many were isolated and had little in common with their fellows, except a label. Grace had no real friends within the institution.

> I wasn't bothered really. I hadn't any (friends) really. I just sat on my own doing me fancy work and me knitting.

Joe also kept himself to himself.

> I didn't bother so much about the others at all. I used to go about and keep me mouth shut.

However, there was one sort of relationship that the institution was only too keen to promote: this was the relationship between the more dependent resident and the more able-bodied. The function of the 'high-grade' resident was to promote the smooth running of the institution and what could promote it better than to allocate the care of a highly dependent person to another able-bodied resident. There is no doubt that such enforced relationships could provide people with a focus for their unfulfilled needs for affection and attention. Grace's sister gave birth to a child with severe physical handicaps and Grace, being the child's aunt, was allocated the responsibility of caring for her.

> She (sister) had a miscarriage at first, and then she had this baby. When she had it, it must have touched the baby's brain. It was a lovely baby, it had a big lump on her back. She kept it for three years nearly, before she put her in the colony. She only put her in the colony because she knew I were there and she knew that I should look after her. She were only twenty-one when she died. I used to go up every night to see her — put her to bed.

Grace developed a genuine affection, not only for her niece, but for other people in the same position.

> Villa 6s, it's a heartbreaking villa. I loved it. I loved them. I used to go to villa 2, I loved that one. I didn't mind that they had to be looked after, poor devils. There were some lovely ones. Take them t' toilet and change them. If you took to one and you wanted to keep her and you loved her and then you could be with her all the time.

Grace had much love to offer those she cared for, but such a system was not the result of choice, but of necessity. The recipients of such care had to rely on the integrity of their fellow residents. For some of these helpers, the opportunity to vent their pent-up frustrations, through exploitation, bullying, or abusing dependent residents, must have been hard to resist.

> Knowing the kind of patients who couldn't do certain things for themselves, there were other patients on the brighter side, including myself at the time. If they were asked to do certain things by way of helping the patients and staff, some were ready and willing enough to do it. There were certain grumblesome ones. There were ones who made their feelings felt by being rough with the less fortunate ones. Roughly handling them in the way they went about the job they were meant to do. I was among the ones who did anything I was asked to do 'cos I was able to walk then.

Ernest found himself in the position of having to be helped by other people, but accepted this change in role philosophically.

> There were some (staff) who were a bit on the rough side compared to what they're like at the present time. Needless to say, I'm grateful for those who do help me in those ways (i.e. getting around, toileting, eating, etc.), members of our staff and Muriel. If they happen to be attending another patient, I just wait till they get round to me. If they take more time I'm just patient. I'm able to hold on to my gift of patience! Others get upset and make their impatience known by complaining to the staff supposed to be attending to him. Needless to say, they've ended themselves in trouble and seen the doctor. Lost for a period of time their privileges and conduct money.

Relationships with staff varied greatly. Staff held the keys, literally, to all privileges, to food and drink, to work, rest and play. Some nurses were able to cope with this powerful position and yet remain human and approachable.

> They were all different nurses on every villa. Some were nicer than the others. (On my villa) there used to be a Sister — she was nice, right tall.

Some people, like Elizabeth, were able to develop long-term friendships with some members of staff.

> She were right friendly. She sends me a card for me birthday. She sent me two handkerchiefs and a card.

Violet's only relationship was with her favourite member of staff.

> One, one friend and that were Sister Smith, but when she left. . .

Ernest, the keen observer of behaviour, recognised that the way to develop good relationships with staff was through politeness and obedience.

> They were towards us depending very much on how we behaved. For the most part we got on all right with them. If we behaved well we were treated well. If anything out of the ordinary which didn't do well, we were treated accordingly, according to the offence committed, whatever it was.

The more able a resident was, the more likely he or she was to be valued and appreciated by staff.

> The ones that were able to do things for them; staff enjoyed their being helpful to the less fortunate ones.

For Ernest, relationships with staff were based on an acknowledgement that staff knew best and were in charge. It was not the resident's place to challenge staff authority:

> There were some who used to fight with the staff. The staff used to keep them as best they could. They used to tell them about their behaviour at certain times of the day, bedtimes and mealtimes. How they should behave at the table. I was treated well. The other patients used to speak about them in that way through their own dislike for the members of staff. . . but not in the presence of the staff concerned.

All situations where able-bodied staff care for less able people inevitably attract those who enjoy and exploit the controlling aspects of the caring relationship. Enclosed institutions were specifically designed to exert control. It is not surprising, then, that most people have memories of cruelty and injustice.

> They were strict, though. If others didn't do as they were told, they used to tell them to put them to bed without (any supper), if they didn't do as they were told. They used to try and take them upstairs to bed, make sure they get in and take their clothes away. They didn't do it every time, you know, being nasty. If you didn't do as you were told they'd give you the treatment. (Horace and Henry)

> She was a twister! She twisted the money, fiddled it. They used to kick the patients about. Kick 'em; give 'em stick 'n that, bang 'em about! It was what the staff did. I were on 13 then. There were some that were all right, but there were some bad buggers in there, knocked the patients about! (Joe)

> Mrs Brown, she used to be awful, her. You did anything wrong — God help you! (Grace)

> There were some nasty nurses what used to work there. We're only human, but they were cruel! They used to bray people, sometimes for nothing. It were terrible, the poor lasses were really punished. (Grace)

The doctors were part of this system, for they had been responsible with the Executive Officer for committing people to the institution in the first place. Inside the institution, although viewed with awe, they were, with one notable exception, regarded more as prison governors than as doctors.

> Couldn't speak to girls — 'cos Dr Black wouldn't allow it. (Tom)

> There was Dr Charles, who was one of the strict ones. Before he came here,

he was a prison doctor, which accounted for his strictness in dealing with the patients. (Ernest)

> He were awful, I didn't care for him at all. He were awful, I didn't take any notice of him. He were right funny, he were. (Joe)

> There was one doctor I didn't like, Dr Roberts. He took me to one side and he said it were through me that me mother died. I mean I did me punishment for what I did. (Elizabeth)

The exception, a doctor employed to take responsibility for the physical aspects of medical care, is remembered by all with affection and regard. Joe remembers that Dr Harris had time to listen and would have helped him, had he been able.

> Dr Harris would come round and have a good talk with you, and he'd listen to me and have a good talk. So I'd have a good talk to him about me going out. He told me he'd let me go, and then he died. I had to wait still longer then. (Joe)

Residents were aware of clashes of medical opinion. Dr Harris seems to have had little influence with his colleagues and his humane views clashed with those of the institution's traditions.

> Well, Dr Harris couldn't get what he wanted for us girls and Dr Black wouldn't let him have it. He thought it was rotten. He said it was just like a locked jail and it wasn't for us, that place. (Grace)

His early death must have been a severe blow to many.

Of course, the whole purpose of the institution was to regulate contact between the sexes. The institution had to segregate, control and repress if it was to succeed in its prime purpose of preventing people with mental handicaps 'repeating their type'. The rules were strict, but the reasons for them were neither understood nor accepted by any of the residents. Margaret and Tom recalled those days vividly.

> We never used to talk to men in them days. Daren't even speak to them when we used to go to school. Don't know why. The girls were on one side and the boys were on the other side. We daren't even talk to them. Daren't even look at them! I think we just might get into trouble or something from 'teacher who used to be in 'school. Things have changed a lot since then. Well you can talk to 'boys. Sometimes I was too shy to talk to them. (Margaret)

> Just have a dance on our own. They didn't allow us with the girls. I don't think that was fair at all. Couldn't speak to girls 'cos Dr Black wouldn't allow it. (Tom)

Ernest, who had accepted so many of the institution's other practices, bitterly resented these strictures.

> We weren't able to mix with any of the female patients even if we had anyone amongst them. One or two had girlfriends but weren't able to spend time with them as we are at the present time. We were never told the reason for it. I didn't see any reason for it at all. I just didn't see any reason for it. (Ernest)

> You couldn't mix together as you were able to do in these times. If you have any communication with the girls, it resulted in the person going before one of the senior physicians and losing our privileges and money which we got on a Friday. (Ernest)

> All the girls used to have to sit on one side. You couldn't go near the boys. They were watching you. You were even watched when you went to dances or anywhere. I used to dance with them now and again but I never had a boyfriend. I wasn't bothered 'cos I didn't want men 'cos I'm not very fond but I felt sorry for 'other girls. (Grace)

Some like Grace, quoted above, were not really interested in the opposite sex but still felt keenly the effects of the regime. Others, like David, learned that girls were trouble and it was best to keep away from them.

> No good bothering wi' girls. You'd talk to them but you don't bother with them. You'd get in trouble don't you. I mean you get into trouble bothering with them don't you. I used to talk to them.
> You don't sit with them do you. You sit on one side don't you. You'd get into trouble if you sat wi' girls. Boys have to sit on one side and girls the other, haven't they — get into trouble — play hell with you. (David)

Henry felt the same.

> If you make friends with one (a girl) and they stop with you, they go on to another. 'You can't have him' and she says, 'I'm just having him' and that's how fights are caused. I just walked away and ignored them!

For Elizabeth grief at the death of her boyfriend and the circumstances of her institutionalisation seems to have quelled her feelings for the opposite sex.

> I didn't bother wi' lads then. Not here anyway. Mine was a soldier and he got killed.

The existence and close proximity of large numbers of healthy young men and women stimulated some ingenious ways of circumventing the rules. Grace remembered that cabbages were put to very good use.

> I did cabbage you see. And love letters were sent through cabbages; used to fold them up. They used to cut 'em in half, cabbages, and stick it together again. And when 'boys came in with their pot of tea in a morning, there used to always be a letter underneath. They could've got on bloomin' villa 8 (punishment villa) for months and months if they were found out. They used to say, 'Don't tell 'em.' and I never told, poor lasses. One man there he would never give them boys away. He was ever so good.
>
> They could (shout to each other) near 'kitchen. They used to say, I'll see you later'. I said, 'You won't see me, you might see your girlfriend but you won't see me!'

The consequences of being caught were, for some, an anxiety which diminished enjoyment.

> If you wanted to have a word with them, you used to shout from one villa to 'next. Stand at the corner of your villa and they'd stand at the corner of their villa and shout to one another. If Dr Black or Matron or any of them came, they'd bang you straight to 'office. Put you in a side-room for punishment. (Elizabeth)

> Well, I didn't used to talk to them (lads). I remember when I saw staff pulling her ears. I used to say, 'I'm off! There's staff there looking out. I'm going inside.' (Elizabeth)

For others, this danger just added further spice to beating the system.

> They used to sneak behind... Had to tell 'nurses going for a walk at night. She used to say, 'Be back for so-and-so time,' and they used to go out together. (Elizabeth)

> Some old lads used to go round here to meet women, under this passage, when it was quiet at 'mansion. Get caught by the Matron or Sister, you've had it. You'd get punished. You got punished by 'staff on 'villa. Used to hit 'em, belt 'em! (Frank)

> The only time I've worked with women were in the kitchen. A lot of good laughs wi' em! (Frank)

Despite the institution's strenuous attempts to deny and repress sexual feelings, a few people did develop lasting relationships. Horace had a girlfriend who worked in the laundry; although they do not seem to have had a sexual, or very equal, relationship, nevertheless, the fact that there was one person who cared for him in this way must have helped to make institutional life more tolerable for Horace.

> I had a girlfriend at The Park, but she's not there now. She died. I'd see her every Sunday afternoon in church, then see her again when we used to have pictures. Just Laurel and Hardy and all them. Then I used to see her in dances. Then she worked in 'laundry. I saw her then, kept seeing her then. She used to say, 'Morning, darling, still love me? Give us a kiss.' I give her a kiss and she give me one. She used to put things in me pocket. Cigs she used to give me.
> Girls we used to go out with used to be all right. They've got out now but we haven't bothered since.

Grace, whilst not being interested in men herself, seems to have taken a great deal of interest in the affairs going on around her.

> Elsie, she had lovely hair. There were a boy on villa 13 thought the world of her. She used to go out to nurses' home and go to 'woods with him. You could then, 'cos you weren't locked in nurses' home. He got her all flowers and all sorts. She used to go down to nurses' home and didn't finish till half nine at night.

Perhaps Grace's reluctance to become involved resulted from her observation of at least one such clandestine affair which ended in tragedy.

> They had to be strict. They were ever so strict when Jane had that baby. It were a man in 'laundry that worked on 'machines. He got her into trouble. We were all sent for to 'villa. Straight on villa 8 she went. It were awful. She went away to have it. They wouldn't have known it were him only he tried to poison himself. You had to be very, very careful!

For Joe, his friendship blossomed and led, many years later, to marriage. Joe, in fact, was in his seventies when he and Mary were finally married and moved into a flat of their own outside the hospital. Ernest, too, has had a long-standing friendship with Muriel, a friendship which has grown and deepened despite the fact that they have never lived together on the same villa. Ernest has written an account of his life in the colony and he has allowed us to quote the following, which illustrates the comfort and solace that this relationship has brought to them both.

> Seventeen years this year when Muriel and I first came together. I can honestly say beyond any shadow of doubt that Muriel is to me everything a

girlfriend should be. In fact, she is in many ways more than just a girlfriend, she is more like a sister to me. Because of the things she's prepared to do by way of being helpful to me, taking into mind my disability, being in the wheelchair. Because of her willingness to do anything I ask her and if she can do anything that is helpful to me. She takes me round to the place where they have the service on a Sunday afternoon and the Tea Room in the hospital grounds.

If the day ever came when Muriel was to go any place from here, for what my life would be without her, it would be as good as at an end. There was a time, not long ago, since she was asked to go to Abbey Grange with some of the others. She had her thoughts on me when she gave her answer to that question; knowing something of how I was feeling, she turned it down.

I am hoping and trusting in God for something greater in the future . . . namely that Muriel and I will one day be joined together in marriage as this is a subject on which many people here at The Park are often asking us about, especially the staff and senior nursing officers, though I've always thought they've meant it jokingly! (From *My Life at The Park*, 1974)

The institution was unable to prevent, despite all its endeavours, the most determined men and women from developing relationships with one another. The majority, however, fell victim to the system. The rules, practices and punishments operated by the institution resulted in isolation, not only from the opposite sex, but also from their fellows and relatives and families. In some instances, men, crowded together and denied access to women, turned to each other for comfort and relief.

Although homosexual relationships, sometimes involving the exploitation of dependency, are known to have flourished, only Frank refers to sexual relationships between men.

> If they got caught, they'd be in right trouble. Put in pyjamas. Worse with a woman. It was a risk! (Frank)

In society at large at that time, homosexuality was treated as a crime; in the institution, although it was not desirable, it was apparently considered preferable to heterosexual relationships!

9

'Half of Me Life's Been Wasted'
Changes and Freedoms

During the first forty years of its life, The Park developed an unchanging routine: the pattern of life was explicit and encompassed within its rules and regulations. The Health Service Act 1948 had created some changes. The colonists had then become in-patients and the colony a hospital. The Mental Health Act 1959 continued the process of very slow change which has steadily gained momentum. Within the past decade, the speed of change has greatly accelerated and has swept aside many of the colony's long-cherished standards. Both men and women live on the same villa and there is much greater recognition of individual needs for dignity and privacy.

> I think it's better now. When it altered they said, 'Go on, you can go on your own now.' I was surprised, I just stood there with me mouth wide open.
> She says, 'You don't wanna think about 'olden days what you used to do.'
> I said, 'I'm used to having somebody with me.'
> 'Them days is gone, get out!'
> So I went out. When I first went out on me own I didn't know where I was going!
> She kept saying, 'You don't have nobody with you now. You can do what you like, you're old enough. You're not tied to us. We don't call you patients now.' I've been right happy since. It's better now than it's ever been.
> (Elizabeth)

Elizabeth, admitted to The Park sixty-three years ago following the birth of her daughter, is now preparing herself to leave permanently and take up a new life. She has seen many changes in The Park and for the past few years has lived in a flat with three other people within the grounds of the hospital. This flat is one of four which were created when a villa was modernised. It is quite small and there is insufficient space for each person to have a separate bedroom, so an area is curtained off to create a private space for each person. Although not ideal, Elizabeth greatly values the privacy this affords and the staff's consideration.

There's no doors downstairs but there's curtains. If anybody is bathing you can see them through the curtain. I don't mind that because you can draw the curtain. You can draw them but you can see them walking past. They don't look in. If they want you to get up in the morning, they just knock on the side of your wall and say 'Are you getting up, breakfast is nearly ready', and I shout through and say, 'I'm getting up now and I'll come to it.'

In 1987, Elizabeth had her first experience of living outside the hospital when she was given the opportunity of sharing a flat with three other people.

I got to have three of them (other residents) with me, I can't live on me own. They won't let me go out on me own in case I take poorly or owt.
   It were in November when we come in. We were pleased when we saw it. Now it's done up we found out it's too small. I can't settle with one of them, other two I can. If I'd 've known beforehand I'd 've said no, I wanted a flat of my own. I didn't know she was going to be as nasty as this. And I didn't know I were gonna sleep in the same bedroom. They all know it's not suitable for two of us to sleep in one room.

Greatly valuing her privacy, Elizabeth could not adapt to sharing a bedroom, especially since the woman she shared with did not also share Elizabeth's standards.

She left the bedroom door open. I got up before anybody came in and shut it after her, I told her about it; she got me that worked up, I were getting mad with meself not her. (I was) getting up every morning and banging it. She heard me one morning, she reckoned to be deaf but she heard me one morning. She flew up in air and she told me she went and told staff about me. I don't know what it were over. But it mattered getting up and leaving doors open. If we had bedroom of us own...She's been like it — you couldn't talk to her proper without she got blazed up. I told them. I told social worker and all that I'm not going to stop where there's two in a bedroom and he says it weren't healthy.
   Her and I couldn't agree. She used to lay the table and bang pots about and chunter away to herself. I've decided — I still want to go back. They said can't you give it another chance and see what she is like, I said no. I can't stick it. She got on me nerves that much, I didn't know what I were doing.

Faced with this, Elizabeth made the decision to come back to The Park to the relative privacy of her flat. This failure of her long-cherished ambition to live outside brought to the forefront of her mind all of the conflicting emotions which she had managed to keep at bay in the institution. Speaking at the time about her decision to return, Elizabeth said:

> I don't know whether I can go back. Not to stay there for good, just go there till summat's done. I can't make me mind up, me mind's all on different things. Sometimes I make it up to go back and other times I. . . I'm unsettled, I've been right upset since I come here! One time I cried and cried me eyes out. It's not that I don't like it where I'm living. The place is all right, it's just because of that (woman) she upsets me. It's me own doing if I go back. I've more friends up there than I have down here.

In the turmoil of wondering whether she would ever be able to live outside The Park, Elizabeth found herself dwelling on past injustices and the reasons for her being forced to spend most of her life in an institution.

> It's better now than it's ever been. Well I think so but sometimes I get this. . . all me past comes when I'm by myself. Me mind wandering. . . what I've been doing, why I shouldn't be here.
>
> Any old nurses will tell you I've been here a long time. I think I should be out now, a home for meself!

With help, Elizabeth is coming to terms with her past and although she is ambivalent about moving out, is now ready to try again. She is realistic about the fact that her sixty years can't simply be wiped out when she leaves.

> I'll miss this place though. I've been here that long time, I can't get used to being anywhere else.

She now has the chance of moving into a private residential home where she will have a room of her own. Having paid a visit, she is reserving her judgement until she has some experience of living there.

> I don't know to tell the truth, you've got to live with them to find out what they're like. I won't know till I've been there but I'm hoping it will be a better place than where I've been. More homely. I'm hoping it will be more pleasant than where I've been. As soon as I got in and looked at it I says. 'I like it.' I didn't say I didn't like it, I just said that I liked it. When I saw just one room, I thought, I'll have a look through the other rooms. They were nearly all the same but I think I'll stick it this time.
>
> It were more bigger than where I've been before. There's more room in it. You can have visitors. If you want to go out, you tell them what time you're going to come in, what time you'll be back. If you've got a TV you can take it with you.

Loneliness is a possibility that Elizabeth has thought about:

Well, I would ask them if I could visit somebody here, not always but just now and again. I could ask if I could have visitors off flat 3 or flat 2. See if I can come up and ask them to come. What will make it worse is that I don't know my way.

Despite her fears and anxieties, after waiting more than sixty years, Elizabeth at the age of eighty-one is determined to prove that she can live outside The Park.

I'm ready to try it again. Social worker says if you don't really like it, you can always tell us — you can stay where you are. I told him I'd try and stick it this time.
I shouldn't really be here. I should be out. I've said this because they've said it. Yes, I shouldn't be here really.

For Ernest, however, the chances of living outside the institution never came. Although more than twenty years younger than Elizabeth, his physical health deteriorated and he relied heavily on staff. Interviewed a few months before his death, he was philosophical about his position. Despite his physical handicaps, some aspects of his life had improved and he, like Elizabeth, greatly valued the staff's consideration of his privacy.

Not like it is now, pretty different in the present day to what it was then. I'm put in a bath now and I just have someone to do the parts that I can't manage myself — round me back — and then left to carry on myself until I'm finished. It's much better now!

His long-standing friendship with Muriel has helped to compensate for many of the privations he has suffered. For him, it was not a question of where he lived, so long as he continued to live near Muriel.

I haven't thought seriously about it (moving out). Having my friend Muriel in mind, if it is possible to go some place together rather than two different places. So long as we can still be together I don't mind what happens, stay here or go elsewhere.
If it happened to be a house where the two of us can be sleeping in different rooms, that would be quite sensible to me. I'd be quite happy about that.

When writing about his life, Ernest's concerns were as much for other people as for himself.

If I had three wishes, the first would be that I could go to the local parish church more often than at present and this on foot rather than in a wheelchair.

My second wish would be that all wheelchairs both in this and other hospitals could be abandoned and those who have to use them be able to walk about and live a normal, healthy life and finally, my third wish would be to spend a holiday from time to time with relatives or friends with whom I've come in contact over the years since I first came into hospital and I have met certain ones who, if they could, would only be too willing to take me in.

I hope very much, by the help of God, and that of the staff, doctors, physiotherapists, etc. . . . that the time will eventually come when I shall be able to abandon the use of the wheelchair completely and be able to walk without any form of support whatsoever. All this will enable me to be more active and be able to be of assistance to other people, doing things for them which they are unable to do for themselves. And finally, I would be able to go places with those of my friends who go out on parole every week, especially with my very dear friend Muriel.' (From *My Life at The Park*, 1974)

Ernest died in The Park in the summer of 1989.

Now totally blind, Frank is forced to depend on other people to help him outside.

> I'm fed up a bit. Don't get out at weekend here. Not so much, don't get out. No-one to go out with you, no staff. And there's no residents what can take you out. I used to go out by meself at one time.

His one outing is to go to the hospital tea room and 'that's not much exciting is it?' After a lifetime of hard work in The Park, Frank, still very independent, is bitter that he is still there after nearly sixty years.

> Dr Black here were awful. I'd have been out before now if it hadn't been for him — 'cos of him. I'd have been out of here. I didn't want to be here. He said I'd have to stop a bit longer. I've stopped here too long!!

Given three wishes, all of them would be 'to be out'.

> Don't want to be here all me life. I've been a good time here — fifty years. They think you're crazy wandering around here. I've been waiting a good long time, haven't I? Sheltered housing would do me wouldn't they? It would be all right for me, with somebody with me. The Sister told me that I've been put forward to go into a house. She said it was very nice. And there's a few more going to the same place that I'm going. But I haven't heard any more since. They keep saying they'd consider it and consider it and find me a place. I don't want to go in an old people's home, I don't want it! I want to settle down in me own place. I want one of these houses what they're putting 'em in. Like sheltered homes out there. I'd have to have someone with me.
>
> There's girls gone out wi' some o' lads at Abbey Grange into the same home as them. It's a good idea, it's sensible. I'd prefer rooms of your own.

> They have rooms of their own when they go out. Not comfortable (here), can't trust a lot of them!

As each year progresses, it will become less and less likely that Frank, now well into his seventies, will have his wish for he is not high on the hospital's list for resettlement into a group home.

Henry and his friend Horace escaped (officially) more than a decade ago. Both left with sighs of relief:

> I didn't used to like it. It were right awful! You couldn't talk to 'females. You couldn't do nowt! Could only talk to friends on your own side and play cards. (Horace)

> You couldn't go to other villas. I didn't like anything! (Henry)

When they left, few, if any, of the present improvements had been made. The villas were still segregated and most of the bureaucratic restrictions were still in force.

> It's all changed. You can go out any time you want now. You can just walk out of the gates now. I couldn't do that before but you can now.'

However, Horace remembers with distaste the work he was forced to do in the colony:

> If somebody messed himself, them that can't help themselves, we used to clean it and bath 'em.

In Henry's view, not all the changes were for the better.

> It's all changed now. You've got men mixed up with ladies. I don't like it. In a way it isn't supposed to be — a lad going into a female's room!

Henry and his friend were among the first to leave whose departure was organised by the institution and the local authority. They left to go and live in a social services hostel and were overjoyed at having been able to make the system work in their favour.

> I'm glad to get out. I was there for forty-eight years. I had to fight myself out! And here I am now — a free man. Best man wins!

Moving out of the institution is, for those with additional physical handicaps, a great deal more uncertain. Ernest did not succeed and Frank may not see hopes achieved. Margaret and Joan, who both rely on wheelchairs for all mobility, also cherish the desire to leave. In their case, age is on their side, as despite the fact that they have had over forty years each in the institution, they are still both in their fifties. They share Elizabeth's and Ernest's appreciation of the changes, particularly greater freedom.

> Now I like it. Now I am a lot happier. I never used to go home or anything. Never used to go home in my life. It's only since I've been on villa 8 that I've been going home. Mind you, I know I only go for the day, 11.30 to 6.00. I'm out for dinner and tea. Now I've started going home I'm a lot happier 'cos my Mum can't get to see me now 'cos she's getting old.

Going home gives Margaret peace of mind. Joan, although she has no family of her own, expresses similar feelings.

> She's happy now 'cos she gets to her friend's home, Rose the cleaner. (Margaret interpreting for Joan)

Improvements not withstanding, they too feel that they have been in The Park for too long.

> It was all right then. I think it was nice and all right. I hadn't been here long enough then, but now I'm thinking I've been at The Park too long now. I wish I could leave in one way. I don't mean to be nasty. I'd like to go and see somewhere, you know, nice places.
>
> You know I'd like a change. But if I did have a change, people who can't walk and have been in a chair... if I did go out of this place altogether, it would have to be somewhere where it's all flat and even, where there's no steps. Would they let us have a change?

Life at The Park is made bearable for those who have friends. Margaret and Joan have been friends since they first met nearly forty years ago. Their friendship is as important to them as leaving.

> I'd feel lost without Joan, not having her to talk to. Without having to talk to each other, I'd feel lonely. I would rather like to be with Joan to help her to talk, to be right helpful like I always have been.
>
> I'm just getting a bit fed up of being here. You know I've been here a long time. Are they supposed to be building some houses? I hope I'm not going to stay here much longer!

George and Tom moved together into a modern flat in a popular village some miles from the hospital three years ago. George's physical handicaps mean that he has to use a wheelchair. His friend Tom helps him and both are determined to prove their independence. After living in the flat for a few weeks, they decided they no longer needed to have staff on duty at night. When asked what they remembered best about The Park in the old days, they were unanimous that what was best was being able to escape.

> Going out on trips.

George has never settled in The Park. Whilst there he constantly pestered the doctors, psychologists and social workers with requests for a change. He had always wanted to leave. Now both he and Tom are content with their life but they do miss some of their friends who still live at The Park. Asked if they would like to return, they were both adamant:

> No I would not. 'Cos you've got freedom. Go out on your own.

Joe left the institution with his wife Mary to live in a flat. Sadly Joe died about a year ago but he did realise both of his ambitions. Admitted when he was nine, he remembers his mother's visits and her advice:

> Before me mother died, she told me to get married. That was her wish, so I did her will.

The death of Dr Harris meant that he had to wait until he was seventy-two before he left the hospital.

> Dr Harris would come round and have a good talk to you and he'd listen to me and have a good talk about. . . So I'd have a good talk to him about me going out. So he told me he'd let me go, so, and he died. I had to wait then longer still.
>
> Ah yes, I waited for the opportunity I had to get out.

To be successful, it was important to win the good opinion of the staff.

> They take my character. . . so I got round him like and was happy to tell him about these here flats. 'Cos I wanted to go in one. So he told me I had to wait a bit. He said he would put me down for Abbey Grange, so as soon as there was two beds spare me and her went down there. After I'd been down at Abbey Grange for a bit, I saw the charge nurse and I shut 'door and asked him if I could have a flat and he said yes, and I did. I told him I wanted a flat just like that, so John said to me, 'I'll get you one but you will have to wait a long time.' I only waited a year and he took me up here to have a look at it.
>
> After all this I've settled down here now and I don't want to move out. A person asked me about moving out of here, so I said, 'No, I've bought

everything, carpets, curtains and all 'lot and I weren't moving out of here at all.

Joe continued to live in his flat with Mary his wife until he became seriously ill when hospice care was arranged for him. Following his death, his wife gave up the flat and now lives in a residential home.

Sally was a close friend of Joe and Mary and moved out with them to the same block of flats. For her, it was her third attempt to live outside.

> I thought I'd get out. I got out with my mother at first. Then she died and I had to go back. I were in the same room with her and our Pauline, that's me brother's wife, she fetched us a cup of tea. I said to me Mam, 'Mam, are you going to drink your tea?' — and there was no answer. She were gone. I went into hysterics. They gave me a cigarette to bring me round. They said I'd have to go back to 'Park 'cos I couldn't stop at home on me own. Me brother couldn't take me, he said there were nobody there 'cos they were both out working. There were nowhere to stop so I had to come back.

Her second attempt was successful for a time.

> I was at Brighton for five years. Taking bagwash to laundry and shopping and looking after five children. Some neighbours wrote a letter to Dr Black and told them they were no relations to me. So I had to come back.

Sally hated life in The Park.

> I kept running away. I got fed up, it used to drive me crazy. I used to do stupid things to myself — cut myself. Nearly cut one of my arteries, nearly was a goner.

Eventually, she learnt to tolerate, if not to accept it. On 24 June 1966 she was given a letter by Matron, the contents of which were to be 'personally explained to her'. This letter was written by the Medical Superintendent and said:

> Patients admitted informally are not subject to detention. Whilst in hospital they are expected to co-operate with the medical and nursing staff and accept any rules and restrictions thought to be necessary in their own interests or in the interests of others.
>
> Patients who wish to leave. . . are strongly advised to discuss this in advance with the hospital doctor. . . Patients will normally be allowed to leave. . . In exceptional cases, it may be found necessary to take steps to authorise patients' detention under the procedures laid down in the Mental Health Act 1959.

This letter may have been read out to her at the time but the legal language was not easily comprehended by people unused to receiving any written communications. She remembers nothing of it being explained to her but she had preserved the letter carefully and when its contents was explained to her twenty-three years later, she commented that nobody had told her.

> Nobody — until you told me. I got it when my mother were living.

Resigned to life in the institution, Sally set about getting herself out by different means.

> I were good to staff. When they used to come on duty, used to get up and make them a pot of tea, put it on a tray for them and cups and saucers and take it into the office to them. That's how I got a good name.
> They give me a good name, that's how I got out. I felt right chuffed! If I'd 've stopped at The Park I'd 've been killed! Half me life's been wasted!

Leaving became more important as time went on. As the more able people left or were moved to other villas, life became duller.

> We had to make ourselves jolly if we could. But if you got mixed up with the mad ones, you couldn't have much fun. At mischievous day I once tied a chamber on a string on 'bed. When they went to bed, chambers were rattling. We used to put sweeping brushes in and chamberpots. That were fun. But it went completely when all others went, all the good ones. They all went and left us. So we had no fun at all.

From The Park, Sally was transferred to the Abbey where she was taught to cook.

> Then I did so well, they let me out. I were very pleased.

Sally moved out five years ago. She was to move into a downstairs flat with a friend but before the flat became available, this plan had to be changed.

> I was supposed to be having somebody in but that girl died. They called her Mavis. She died, she had a stroke — so I had to go in on my own.

The area where Sally lives is solidly middle class and respectable. Her flat is modern and well appointed but the neighbourhood has suffered from a spate of burglaries. Knowing this, Sally was understandably apprehensive:

It were all right but there were some robbers went downstairs to the other lady's house. They took all her jewellery and all her food. She'd been robbed three times. Before I went in that flat robbers had been in there. I were frightened of that. I said I didn't want to stop. So they got me this flat. Well I get a bit frightened here on my own.

Since moving, Sally, who makes friends readily, has found that her circle of friends and acquaintances has greatly decreased. The first and most important loss was the death of her friend Joe.

She got me this flat to look after Joe and Mary and then Joe went, I never felt the same. That's two shocks I've had — me mother's death and Joe's death.

Despite these bereavements, Sally has been determined not to succumb to self pity but to try her best to help those around her.

Mrs Wilson who lived at bottom had all locks on her windows but they don't put them in upstairs, only downstairs. That lady's died now. She used to have a home help 'cos she had a bad heart. She fell down and broke her hip and they took her to hospital and she were never right since. They had to feed her with a drip and she wouldn't eat. She were eighty-two. She were right good to me. I used to do messages for her. You know, go for her prescriptions to the doctor. She once asked me if I would stop with her all night. She said, 'You can sleep with me.' I wanted to go back in me own flat. I used to go and talk to her. When I talked with her, I left her and she were all right.

Her daughter rung me up and asked if I'd stop with her while ambulance came for her because she fell down and cut all her head at the back. When ambulance men came, she asked them if I could go with her to hospital. They said, 'No, there were no need.' They said she would be all right. She never knew she had cut her head till I noticed it.

Sally takes great pride in her flat which is sparkling clean but she feels lonely after sharing her life with so many people for so long.

I miss all my friends up there. I used to have a lot of friends.

She still has contact with Joe's wife Mary.

Social worker asked me once if I wanted to go to an old people's home, I said no. I think she wanted me to go there because Mary was there. Nobody bothers with her. Because I were her friend, I used to look after her and her husband. When I go to see her, she goes, 'When are you coming again, Sally? I miss you. I don't like it here.' It's because they make her do things. When she were in the flat, she wouldn't do anything, the home help used to tell her to do things. She got mad with her and kicked her on the leg. She said, 'What do you come here for, we can do it on us own. We don't want you.' But Joe liked her, liked home help. When we went to Scarborough, he bought her a watch.

Visits to friends who live some distance away pose problems.

I can't find it. Social worker took me there but she's that busy, she can't do it so much.

Sally has little confidence in her ability to travel alone. She would like to go back to the 'over sixties club' at The Park to visit her friends but:

You see I get all mixed up with the buses. When I go to my brother's I sometimes get the wrong bus. Then I get off and I lose me way. Then I get lost, I get frightened. I have to ask somebody where I am.
When I were on holiday I got lost. I had to ask somebody and he said just go up that hill and you'll find it and I did. I were all on me own. I went right down the hill to the shops, that's when I got lost. The lady at the hotel kept telling me to go out, so I went out. She said go out for some fresh air, so I did.
I used to have a friend to go out with but she packed me up. She got jealous because I were stopping with another lady, at her house for the weekend. She got funny about it. She just packed me up, she never came no more. So that were that.'

Having someone to share her flat does not seem to be possible.

There's only one bedroom, I don't think they'll allow it. You can't even have pets.'

She would like to live in a group home with two or three others with staff to look after her. In the meantime, the burden of loneliness is alleviated by the Social Services Family Placement Scheme. Sally goes:

Every four months for a fortnight. I pay for it meself, sixty something. I go out shopping with her, there's shops all there. She took me to the park with the two boys. They were playing football. I enjoyed it. I did me best. She asked me if I enjoyed it. I said yes.
At first, I went for a week and social worker asked me how I liked it. I said, 'Oh, I like it very much,' and she asked if I wanted to go for a fortnight and I said yes. You see you've got somebody there to talk to.
She's putting me into another bedroom next time I go — a right posh one.

Grace also lives on her own in a flat. Her first small taste of dignity and self-esteem amazed her:

Then they allowed us to go outside with us visitors. That shocked me, my goodness!

Then we got lovely dresses from 'sewing room and we looked right nice at visiting time. We looked different girls with shoes on 'n all!

Grace has been living in her flat for many years and she recalls the hearing which eventually agreed to her discharge.

It were some big man up from London that sent for me. Said that I shouldn't be in there. There were a lot of girls that shouldn't 've been in. If you could get up at five o'clock in the morning, clean a boiler, you're not 'mental' if you can do that. Mind you, there were trouble when they saw that I did it. It weren't allowed, it weren't a girl's place. But we had to do, there were nothing else.

One o' men said, 'Grace's getting right awful, she's fed up, she wants to go out. Committee come and doctor come. I was dressed nice, put a nice dress on. Made cups of tea for 'em and they said I shouldn't be here. I was out before I knew where I were. I was happy as anything! I knew I'd do it!

Social Services came to see me about three weeks ago and said, 'You are marvellous, Grace! You've done well!' I don't have any men in my flat or lodgers.

When I went up t' garden party up there, they've altered it. Not many girls that I know there now. They've all gone. I'm living them out.

It's altered a lot since I've been there. Them villas look beautiful. If they close it down they've wasted their money 'cos they've done it marvellous.

I can make me own Yorkshire puddings better than what they can! There again I never saw bloomin' Yorkshire puddings! Bloomin' rice pudding were like water! You couldn't have extra, not like now, I make what I want!'

Living alone after thirty-three years of institutional life has been highly successful for Grace.

I wasn't old, were nearly fifty when I left. I couldn't believe it that I'd got this flat. He said, 'We'll go down for it this afternoon.' I just couldn't believe it! You didn't learn as much to come out into freedom. Me mother used to help me do a lot of things.

Hard working Doris, who took such a pride in her work, left the institution only a few months ago. Like everyone else she has appreciated the changes in The Park.

Well you have it more to yourself. It's quiet, you haven't the noise. There were noise all the time; you couldn't get out of it at The Park. It's a mad place now. We all call it 'Mad House. Before we come away it were 'Mad House with all the windows and doors breaking it up.

Doris and a small group of her friends were identified for discharge into the community in 1984. She moved with them into Abbey Grange in 1986 so that they could learn more domestic skills. Doris has had a very long wait for her flat. She reconciled herself to this and despite fifty-two years of institutional life, nevertheless, she is able to judge other people's needs as being more pressing than her own.

> Well, there's no houses to get. Wanted something flat, like the hall without the steps, but there doesn't seem to be any. I mean all I do is look. We haven't to worry about any of it. But there's a lot of young ones waiting for houses and it's just 'same for old ones and lame ones, they don't want any steps.

Eventually in November 1988 she and one of her friends moved into a residential home. Each was to have had a separate bedroom but they decided to share one and use the other as a private sitting room.

> It's all right like that. You could have one of your own of you wanted but we said we wanted two together. Two beds in one room. I think it's better like that. We've known each other a long time in The Park.

For Doris the move is proving a definite change for the better. She began to find that life in Abbey Grange had become quite disturbed.

> It's all right here. Well just at first, you had to get used to it. It's all right now. We thought we wouldn't like it with having been in Abbey Grange so long. It was a nice house, a big house when we first went but it isn't now. You see, they've got a whole lot of boys in, a whole lot from The Park and it isn't nice now. There's a lot moved out now. They spoilt it, you know, getting all that lot in.

Where she lives now is very close to the place she used to live before she came into The Park.

> I don't know my way now. I used to live here in 1917. I knew the farm, a nice farm. Go for milk and eggs. All fields, haymaking. I knew all the shops and the way to the park. I don't know my way now. You see it's all altered. You have to get somebody to go with you and show you where it is now. It's all altered. I was only a girl then.

Doris and her friend greatly appreciate the quality of the food in her new home.

> Good food, just like you get at home. All good stuff. It's done right you know, Yorkshire puddings and meat and that. You get some nice food here.

You didn't at The Park, oh it was — you couldn't eat it. All mixed up like that so you didn't know what you were eating.

Doris finds the other residents friendly and she is shortly to be joined by one of her old friends Elsie. In fact she has only one complaint about her new life: in Abbey Grange she and her friends were able to go out regularly to the local shops, now she doesn't know her way and has not yet found anybody to take her.

We used to go down to the shops a few times, me and Dot and Etty and Carrie. Many a time when we wanted things. We used to go to the Post Office like and used to go for a walk. You see there's nobody here to go with. Some will fetch you things but nobody to take us like.

Of the seventeen people who began this project three years ago, four have since died. Violet and Enid died before they had any chance to live again outside The Park. Ernest died, accepting his situation but nevertheless still clinging to the hope that he and Muriel would one day marry. Frank's wish to move is tinged with desperation. For Joan and Margaret, the intensity of their feelings about still having to live in The Park is offset by having close personal friends.

Nine people now live in the community. Elizabeth, Doris and Elsie are just beginning their new lives. For Joe and his wife, marriage and a home of their own outside The Park was the fulfilment of a lifetime's ambition. Grace is proud of living alone but for Sally the experience is marred by loneliness. For Tom and George and Henry and Horace, living outside the hospital with their friends is a rewarding and satisfying experience.

10

'It's All Changed'

In the preceding chapters, the history of one institution for people who were labelled mentally defective has been recounted through the reminiscences of seventeen of its inmates. These seventeen people are survivors: they have endured a lifetime of being forcibly segregated from family, friends and once-familiar places. Each has coped with the institution's official and unofficial rules, customs and practices through rebellion or passivity, acquiescence or determination. Each set about coping with the dull uniformity imposed on them: some have fallen in love, despite the obstacles put in their way; many have taken a great deal of pride in their work; others, in despair, have run away and enjoyed a temporary, illegal freedom; some set about making friends of the staff; others made friends with religion. Above all, throughout their stay, they have had faith in the belief that ultimately, through hard work and good behaviour, they would be rewarded with a place in the outside world. Four will now never achieve that aim; four are still waiting to be selected for resettlement, increasing age and physical disability decreasing their chances of success.

Because these men and women were among the most able, 'the high grades' in the institution, they were the most able to manipulate the rules to their advantage and, within the confines of the colony, they had more opportunities to express their own needs and develop self-respect and personal status. What about the lives of their less able colleagues, 'the low grades', those who are unable to speak for themselves? In 1982, there were approximately 150 people who were unable to speak, see, hear and/or look after their own physical needs. It is unlikely that there has ever been fewer than this number since the extensions were built in the 1940s. The 'lowest grades' were isolated even within the institution itself. Segregated from their more able colleagues in buildings on the edge of the campus, as far away from public eyes as possible, their lives must have been unremittingly boring: no work, no education, no stimulation. Dressed, washed and fed by overworked, often untrained orderlies and overworked, untrained and sometimes resentful inmates, their lives were, at times, distressingly uncomfortable. Epileptic fits, enemas, drugs, a lack of basic physical aids and, amongst staff generally, a lack of knowledge about preventing physical deterioration and deformity, coupled with an inability on the residents' part to communicate with or to influence those around them, must have been, for many of the most disabled patients, a living nightmare. For this group of people, change has been very slow. As recently as 1978, Maureen Oswin in her book *Children Living in Long Stay Hospitals*[1] observed and recorded the unwitting cruelty and deprivation of institutional care for the most severely handicapped. Mrs Oswin was, moreover, describing an improved life-style, for by this time all children, irrespective of handicap, were educated in school. So the children at least received a change of environment and stimulation. Although a few of the most severely handicapped people are now living in small group homes, the majority are left behind or left till last if institutions are being run down and closed.

It is small wonder then that being acknowledged as a 'high grade' was very important to residents for it had major consequences for an individual's quality of life within the institution. As Grace put it,

> When they found out I were higher grade, then you got a bit more privileges to what the others did. You could do more you see.

At the same time, she and the others deplored the use of these and other terms, not only 'high' and 'low grade', but also 'idiot', 'imbecile', 'feeble-minded', 'mentally defective' and 'mental handicap'.

Frank described them as:

> Terrible words! I didn't like them. Not nice words to talk to people.

For Ernest, such terms were inhumane and degrading and he was very aware of the effect that such terms had on people.

> I didn't like that way of putting it. I was told I was one of the brighter ones, which is true. In many ways, I was able to do things the less fortunate ones haven't been able to do. I didn't like that way of describing anyone. I can't really find the words to describe. . . I felt really bad about it. I've actually heard patients being called by the names you've used by members of staff, just call them an idiot or things like that. I think it did used to (upset people) because the patients referred to in that way used to speak rottenly of the staff who spoke to them in that way — but not in the presence of the staff concerned.

All felt that such terms implied that they were somehow to blame for their handicap.

> They used to call them 'low grades'. They should never be called 'low

[1] Oswin, M *Children Living in Long Stay Hospitals* Heinemann Medical, 1978

grades', when they're not fit to do anything with their self, should be called, 'they can't help it'!

Grace further pointed out the effects that such terminology has on the way staff think about the people they are supposed to be looking after.

> It were a mental hospital. Nobody can help being backward. It's not our fault! Why should people mock people? It isn't their fault that they're like that. Some staff thought they were clever, but they weren't! They were there to help us, not to put us down! Some of them people couldn't walk hardly. They (staff) used to mock 'em. They were there to help 'em!

Terminology such as 'imbecile' and 'idiot', 'high' and 'low grade' is no longer officially used. Modern terms are 'mental handicap' and 'learning disability'. Very few people now believe mental handicap to be a major social evil and the cause of most of the crime, immorality and poverty in the world.

Although people are no longer officially assessed and certified as mentally deficient and incarcerated in institutions, assessment and classification are still the mainstay of the caring system. Just as Elizabeth, Joe and David were required to perform to a certain standard on tests of intelligence in the 1920s and were institutionalised when they failed to reach this standard, so now developmental assessments, intelligence tests and assessments of daily living skills are used to determine which service people receive, which school they attend, who they live with and where they live. Having the 'wrong' IQ can still prejudice access to general medical and psychiatric services and general education.

Nowadays assessments are much more related to the skills needed in everyday life in the community and are of undoubted value in identifying the skills people need to manage their own lives. Nonetheless, the principal way in which assessments are used, particularly when they are used with adults, remains essentially to exclude. Joe, Grace and Sally were able to impress staff with their skills; Joe's expression 'they take my character' summarises this process of selection. Formal assessment and informal opinion and prejudice were the basis on which people were certified and admitted to the colony. Such formal and informal assessments are now employed to decide which people should leave the hospital and be resettled into the community. Those who do not do well according to such assessments are not usually considered for resettlement. Frank and Ernest were for many years valued workers. Frank made mattresses and doormats and worked as a domestic for the staff and Ernest worked as a tailor. Ernest retired because of increasing ill health, a fact which meant that, able though he was, he would no longer be high on the priority list for living in the community. In fact, he died, still living in The Park, just before this book was finished. Frank's blindness and increasing ill health jeopardize his chances too. Ironically, despite being classed for many years as the most able of the 'high grades', he now fails to meet the new criteria. Frank is particularly bitter about his powerlessness to effect any change.

> They keep saying they'd consider it and consider it and find me a place. I don't want to go in an old people's home. I don't want it! I want to settle down in me own place! I want one of these houses what they're putting 'em in. Like sheltered homes out there. I'd have to have someone with me.

The destiny of those who remain is still controlled by staff. 'They' say who will live where and when and, often, with whom.

The majority of people whose histories have been recorded here feel that there have been changes for the better. They can go out by themselves: they can visit relatives and friends; men and women live in the same villa and a lucky few even have their own bedroom. They no longer have to have institutional clothing but choose and buy their own. Many more people go on holiday, some to exotic places. There is a greater appreciation of the need for privacy and a more widespread acknowledgement of individual needs and wishes. They have, undoubtedly, benefited from greater freedom and progress.

But beneath this veneer of greater freedom for the more able residents, better furniture, better clothes and nicer surroundings, many of the fundamental attitudes and prejudices which led originally to the establishment of colonies remain virtually untouched. Assessment and classification still abound. So too does arbitrary removal from home, whether this home is with family or friends or is a group home, hostel or hospital. When relatives die or carers can longer care, sons and daughters are fitted into vacancies wherever these happen to be. Just as the inmates were forced to fit into the colony, so today people have to accommodate to available places. If they do not fit in or object to their placement, the label 'behaviour problem' is likely to be applied. Services are simply not financed to meet individual needs, nor maintain more than a handful of people in their local community. Sudden removal from familiar faces and places for those who have spent many years living at home is a common experience. Many are truly 'sans everything' if their carers die. Rehabilitation systems often involve people moving, whether they will or not, through two, three or even more 'homes'. Individual needs come a very poor third to expediency and economy which are as much a motivation for the present system as they were for the original establishment of the colony.

Colonies deliberately exploited their workforces of able-bodied residents. It made economic sense to do so. Many of these people were taught useful skills such as farming, market gardening, tailoring, laundry work, domestic work and so on. These skills were largely employed within the institution and without pay. After the Mental Health Act 1959, many of the able-bodied were free to leave. The Park hospital's population declined by a hundred in the ten years following the Mental Health Act. Since admission and death rates matched one another, this did represent a significant loss to the economy of the hospital. The hospital began to employ domestics, house-mothers and other staff, and residents were no longer an important part of the workforce by the mid-1970s. Instead, they were occupied in various ways such as craft, woodwork and art. The concept of teaching practical work skills was no longer a prime concern. The colony had not paid its certified workers for work which was a duty and also perhaps a penance. Today, the efforts of people with a mental handicap are still largely unrecognized and unvalued. Goods are often sold for the cost of the materials only. Packing or small assembly work is rewarded with token pay of somewhat less than £6 per week. In many places, this 'pay' is still at the discretion of the staff and can be withdrawn for infringement of rules, irrespective of the amount of work that has been carried out.

In recent years, however, there has been a greater recognition of the value of one of the major purposes of the earlier colony system, that is, the teaching and utilisation of practical work skills. These are now being developed in ways that should enable people with mental handicap to become valued members of their local community. For example, efforts are being made through the Manpower Services Commission and local enterprises to enable people with handicaps to learn the skills of and be supported in real jobs with proper wages. Colleges of further education are now taking a greater interest in providing courses for people with a mental handicap and education authorities are beginning to implement a policy of integration into local primary and secondary schools. This could herald a real change in the fortunes of people with handicaps, provided there is a corresponding change in government policy about benefits. Too many people fall into the benefits trap. Being unable to earn as much as they could receive in benefits, they work for pocket money or are 'occupied' in training centres. This is no substitute for having a wage packet and the rights, the protection and the responsibilities that are accorded to paid employees.

Within The Park, change has now come full circle. Residents are again encouraged to make beds, do cooking, cleaning and ironing. Each villa is gradually becoming responsible for its own domestic and other chores again and soon it will revert to the situation thirty ago which Margaret remembers.

> We didn't have cleaners them days, they all had to clean their own. They had to clean up after themself, tidy all up, do the washing up.

Now the aim is to enable the residents to learn to be responsible for themselves and to become as independent as possible. It is worth while reflecting that one of the original aims of the institution was 'the formation of habits of cleanliness, self-reliance and discipline'. Whether the present move towards self-sufficiency is truly rehabilitative in intent or, as before, simply economic expediency remains to be seen.

There is now greater public awareness of conditions in long-stay hospitals and other institutions. The various hospital scandals of twenty years ago brought these to public attention. The worst excesses of The Park's system of control are no longer practised but the concepts of care and control, which have dominated the care of people with mental handicaps for more than a century, are not so easily changed. If someone is behaving in a way that causes problems such as screaming or shouting, swearing or running away, the first option is still, as it was in 1930, the loss of privileges. Loss of cigarettes, visits home, money, trips to the pub and holidays are common sanctions. The second option is still medication. Punishment and control are important aspects of care systems today, be they local authority, private, charitable or health service care systems.

Underlying this desire to control through the application of punishment is the belief that people with a mental handicap are not people like ourselves. Care systems rarely acknowledge the emotional needs of people they allegedly care for: emotions such as anger, despair or grief are too often classed as 'naughtiness' and, in many cases, little attempt is made to understand why someone is behaving in a particular way. This was poignantly described by Anne McDonald in her autobiography *Annie's Coming Out*.[2]

> We were not good patients. We cried because we felt abandoned. The nurses didn't know what to do; they didn't know we could feel anguish. The institute had no tally book for broken hearts.

[2] Cossley, R. and McDonald, A. *Annie's Coming Out* Penguin, 1982

Such attitudes lead to brutal treatment. In 1927 Elizabeth was viewed as childish because she cried easily: any possible association between her behaviour and the fact that she was suffering from a bereavement, the loss of her family and a traumatic change of life was not acknowledged. Despite increasing awareness of the needs of handicapped people, there is still a marked reluctance to acknowledge that many of those whom care systems glibly classify as 'behaviour problems' are suffering from loss and lack.

Not surprisingly, many of the people in this study, after a lifetime of experience under this system, find it hard to recall or articulate their feelings. In commenting on painful experiences and deprivations such as admission, lack of personal possessions, birthday celebrations, friendships or visits from relatives, people would say 'I didn't bother', 'I didn't feel anything' or 'a bit fed up'. Ignoring, rejecting or minimising their feelings were ways of coping. This is evidenced in Margaret's description of her reaction as a child when her parents were turned out of the villa for arguing in front of her, 'crying, you know, in my own way — tears'. Inherent difficulties in interpreting and describing feelings may well have been compounded by the fact that the institution neither encouraged nor expected the inmates to need to do so. Pretending not to feel or not to mind must, for some, become an automatic and effective method of coping with the pain of neglect.

As people found that their experiences were valued and were listened to, so they gained in confidence in themselves. Some began to admit to their feelings. All those remaining, without exception, wished to leave: 'I hope I'm not going to stay here much longer.' Those who were still living in The Park expressed their feelings of being stigmatised by the situation. Frank said:

> They think you're crazy wandering around here. They think you're mad in here.

The most obvious change is in the mixing of the sexes on villas. It is no longer accepted that handicapped women are 'twice as prolific' as non-handicapped women. Rigid segregation does seem to be a thing of the past. This does not, however, imply that there is a universal acceptance that people with a mental handicap are adults with rights and responsibilities which may include sexual relationships and marriage. Joe and Mary, with the blessing of staff, married and left the institution. Ernest and Muriel developed a mutual supporting, loving and lasting relationship. These are exceptional. The institution did not encourage friendships of any sort. Recognition of sexuality and preparation for adulthood are not integral parts of the education system in special schools. Female sterilization and the pill are sometimes used as solutions to 'problem relationships'. Friendship and sexual relationships are undoubtedly the most challenging aspect of helping people who may not be wholly independent. In such situations, the power of the care-giver, whether paid staff or relatives, is absolute for they can recognise, encourage and enable the development of social behaviour and friendships or they can neglect, ignore, trivialise or destroy relationships. Such power is taken for granted in any situation where people, be they elderly, physically handicapped, mentally ill or mentally handicapped, are dependent on others for help in coping with the everyday tasks of living. Real progress will be made when people, whatever their needs, are actively involved in the hiring and firing of those who are employed to look after them.

There is no denying, however, that many people who would have been hidden away in institutions are now living in the community. Over the past decade, efforts have been made to promote integration into schools, colleges, housing, leisure and work. Achievements have been made through individual determination and initiative. There is a more widespread recognition of the rights of people with a mental handicap. Advocacy and citizen advocacy schemes have been developed to help people cope with the vested interests of statutory authorities, relatives and private enterprise. Nowadays, almost all staff involved in the care, education and training of people with a mental handicap will be aware of the basic concepts of human rights and individual needs.

All too often, however, such concepts are grafted on to the deep-seated, often unconscious attitudes that have been reflected in the preceding pages. Institutional routines, such as the night staff coming on duty at 8.30 p.m., prevent any 'normalisation' of life-style for many residents, particularly those who have physical handicaps. Ernest, in his last years, had to give up the religious services he conducted on his villa and which meant so much to him because:

> The routine has changed with me and the staff's dealings with me. After tea and they've had their own break, I'm brought down here for getting undressed and toileting to change into my nightclothes and then spend the evening watching television until the night staff come on duty.

Normalisation is the new creed and is widely misunderstood. Residents must now, in accordance with the principle of normalisation, be taken out in small groups or individually. In the absence of additional resources, strict adherence to this principle can mean that people go out even less than before. Frank now finds himself isolated within The Park.

> No-one to go out with you, no staff. And there's no residents that can take you out.

Normalisation is interpreted as 'it's their choice' to do or not to do something and has led to a *laissez-faire* attitude which is now to be found in some day and residential services. This no more respects the needs of the people it purports to help than the old institutionalised control systems. The latter ignored their rights, the former ignores the fact that many people with mental handicap need help to exercise these rights and to recognise and undertake their responsibilities.

Colonies were economic and highly successful in that people stayed there and were out of sight and out of mind. There is now a strong counter-movement against the current policy of institutional closure which is motivated by the old mixture of the desire to protect, the desire to exclude, the desire for 'value for money' and a 'pressing local need'. In this case the local need concerns the lack of quality and quantity of services in the community. Old institutions are being replaced by new.[3] Economies of scale and value for money are yet again in the forefront of planning. One alternative to helping handicapped people live like others in the community that has been suggested by a pressure group opposed to closure is the conversion of The Park into a village community. This sort of 'humane solution' is highly favoured. However, it should not be forgotten that the original Park Colony was a shining example of 'the ideal system'. It was a self-sufficient village inside which those who were able were highly productive. They worked hard for no money, were not free to marry, lived only with 'their own kind' and within the confines of rules established by those in charge for the smooth functioning of communal life. The modern village community is based on essentially the same principles.

For ourselves as authors, listening to the reminiscences and to tape recordings has made us uncomfortably aware of the injustices and inhumanity of institutionalised systems of care. Despite years of working in institutions and despite being, we thought, keenly aware of rights and needs, we have been forced to acknowledge to ourselves the devastating effects of institutional life on just seventeen of the many hundreds of people who have lived there. Since the majority of our contributors were unable to read, we arranged readings of each chapter of the book as it was written. Despite the obvious 'correctness' of this

[3] Wertheimer, A. *Hospital Closures in the Eighties,* CMH, London, 1980

attitude we attempted at first to avoid doing so, rationalising this avoidance to ourselves by claiming that the contributors would be upset by the terminology used and by the content of some of the reminiscences. We discovered that we were in fact protecting ourselves against the effects of the care systems we represent. The contributors too felt, at times, acute distress when listening to each others' reminiscences. As Frank said:

> There are some terrible things in that book — terrible times.

Side by side with this painful awareness, we have also become sensible of their humour, resilience and determination. Far from accepting their lot in life, they recognise its injustices and have eagerly grasped the opportunity to give their view of The Park and its history.

> I just like people to know so they can realise what it was we've had to go through. It's not true what was written down! They did it just to keep us locked up, so that people would think we're mental!

APPENDIX I

The Mental Deficiency Act 1913

The Act was intended to provide for the paternal care and protection of people labelled mentally defective. Arguments that such an Act interfered with the liberty of the subject and could lead to capricious detention without adequate cause were outweighed by the desire to protect society from 'degenerate and wastrel classes'.

Described as 'the charter of a real liberty to the large number of chronic mental defectives',[1] it gave powers of certification and compulsory detention to local authorities who would thereby be able to ameliorate society's neglect and rejection through the provision of supervision, accommodation and training. Its ultimate benefit was that it would prove 'a powerful means of assisting to breed out the hereditary transmission of mental defect by preventing the propagation of a degenerate stock'.

Main Provisions of the 1913 Act

1. It established a Board of Control which was directly responsible to the House of Commons through the Secretary of State and which was to form the basis of a complete and co-ordinated state service for the care and control of the mentally deficient.

2. Local authorities were empowered to co-ordinate the administration of the Act, through the appointment of Authorised Officers (also called Executive Officers), so as to avoid wasteful expenditure of public resources.

3. Local authority Care Committees, which organised domiciliary supervision, were strengthened. Those ascertained as mentally deficient and not living in an institution were visited regularly by Voluntary Visitors who reported to the Committee on each case. The Voluntary Visitor also had a duty to help the defective find work and to report to the Care Committee such cases where it was considered inadvisable for the defective to remain at home.

4. The local authority was endowed with powers of certification,

[1] Wormald, J. and Wormald, S. *A Guide to the Mental Deficiency Act, 1913* King and Son, 1914

compulsory detention and removal from home on the grounds of neglect, cruelty of 'other similar causes'.[2]

Legal Definition of Mental Defect

Those considered most suitable to be dealt with under the Act were children who, having attained the age of seven, were deemed incapable of benefitting from education in special school or class or who were discharged from special school as ineducable before attaining the age of sixteen years. Those who were deemed to be educable in special schools could also be dealt with under the Act if they were unable to earn their own living, manage their own affairs and/or conform to the moral code of the community in which they lived.

The Mental Deficiency Act recognised four categories of defect:

Idiots — persons in whose case there exists mental defectiveness of such a degree that they are unable to guard themselves against common physical dangers.

Imbeciles — persons in whose case there exists mental defectiveness which, though not amounting to idiocy, is yet so pronounced that they are incapable of managing themselves and their affairs, or, in the case of children, of being taught to do so.

Feeble-minded — persons in whose case there exists mental defectiveness which, though not amounting to imbecility, is yet so pronounced that they require care, supervision and control for their own protection or for the protection of others, or, in the case of children, that they appear to be permanently incapable by reason of such defectiveness of receiving proper benefit from the instruction in ordinary schools.

Moral defectives — persons in whose case their exists mental defectiveness coupled with strong vicious or criminal propensities and who require care, supervision and control for the protection of others.

---

[2]Heard, H. *The Diagnosis of Mental Deficiency* Hodder and Stoughton, London, 1930

The Process of Certification and Detention

> CIRCUMSTANCES WHICH RENDER A DEFECTIVE LIABLE TO BE DEALT WITH, UPON PETITION, UNDER THE MENTAL DEFICIENCY ACT, 1913.

1. Where it was considered inadvisable for a mentally deficient person to remain at home, the Care Committee had a duty to inform the Authorised Officer who would petition the local authority for an 'Order Sending a Defective to an Institution'.

> THE MENTAL DEFICIENCY ACT, 1913.
>
> COUNTY BOROUGH OF
>
> Petition for an Order sending a Defective to an Institution ~~or placing him under Guardianship~~, presented by an officer of the Local Authority.

2. Parents could also make applications for their son/daughter to be removed to an institution. Again, the Authorised Officer would be involved in drawing up the Petition.

3. The Petition was accompanied by:

(a) Statement of Particulars which gave basic information about the individual and was signed by the Authorised Officer.

> [Form P3.
>
> COUNTY BOROUGH OF
>
> Statement of Particulars to accompany Petition.

(b) Two medical certificates, both dated within twenty-one days of the Petition which certified that the individual was a fit person to be removed.

(c) Parents' consent in writing.

COUNTY BOROUGH OF

THE MENTAL DEFICIENCY ACT, 1913.

CONSENT OF PARENT OR GUARDIAN TO AN ORDER BEING MADE PLACING A DEFECTIVE IN A CERTIFIED INSTITUTION OR UNDER GUARDIANSHIP.

(d) The Statutory Declaration made before a Justice of the Peace or a Commissioner for Oaths and signed by one of the signatories of the Medical Certificate or staff in the Welfare Department. The Declaration stated the grounds on which the person was to be dealt with under the Act, e.g. neglect, cruelty, no visible means of support, criminal offences, habitual drunkard, pregnant with or having given birth to an illegitimate child and in receipt of poor relief or notified by the education authority.

THE MENTAL DEFICIENCY ACT, 1913.

Form P 6.

COUNTY BOROUGH OF

Statutory Declaration to Accompany Petition.

4. When the above papers were in order and duly signed, a Hearing of the Petition before an approved Justice was arranged in a private room at the Town Hall. The Justice could then sign the order for institutional care or for guardianship or dismiss the Petition.

[Form P 7].

THE MENTAL DEFICIENCY ACT, 1913.

CITY AND COUNTY BOROUGH OF

Order sending a Defective to an Institution ~~or placing him under Guardianship.~~

---

5. When the Order had been signed by the Justice, the Authorised Officer arranged for the conveyance of the patient to the institution cited on the Order within fourteen days of the date of the Order. The original Order and the documents on which it was founded accompanied the patient to the institution.

NOTICE OF ADMISSION.

Date of reception order, the   twenty-first   day of   June   19 27

6. Judicial Orders could be renewed by the Board of Control at the end of one or two years and thereafter at five-yearly intervals. A report would be made by one of the Board's Visitors on the home conditions of the patient's relatives and the patient would be re-examined by the Medical Officer. In most cases, a Continuing Order for Detention for a further five years would be signed.

Form D.3 (Five).

MENTAL DEFICIENCY ACTS, 1913-1938.

ORDER BY BOARD OF CONTROL CONTINUING ORDER OR AUTHORITY FOR DETENTION.

---

7. Parents could request in writing for their son/daughter to be withdrawn from the institution. The Board of Control would again consider the means of care and supervision available and would determine whether or not a patient should continue to be detained. If the Board was satisfied with the relatives' home circumstances, then the patient would be released 'on licence'. If, at any stage, the Voluntary Visitor became dissatisfied with the patient's home circumstances, then the licence could be revoked.

Form L. M.D.

LICENCE FOR A PATIENT TO BE ABSENT FROM AN INSTITUTION OR CERTIFIED HOUSE.

---

8. If the Board felt it was in the patient's best interest that he/she should continue in detention, then a barring certificate was issued which prevented further application for a period of six months.

APPENDIX II
Brief Biographical Details

David Born 1912. Attended special school for six years until he was fifteen years old. Mother, a widow with five children, was unable to care for him. He was admitted in 1929. He worked in the hospital stores and pharmacy for many years until his retirement at the age of seventy-five. He was transferred to Abbey Grange in 1981. He is still awaiting sheltered accommodation.

Doris Born 1907. Attended a private school until the age of ten and then went to the local council school. She left at the age of fourteen. Is able to read and write but was said to be unable to do any housework, except under supervision. Father made application for admission following the death of her mother in 1936. Admitted at the age of twenty-eight. Little official information about her occupation in The Park. Did domestic work. Developed some long-standing friendships and moved with two of her friends to a residential home in 1988 at the age of eighty-one.

Elizabeth Born 1909. Admitted to The Orchards in 1927, three months after the birth of an illegitimate baby. Transferred to The Park in 1932. Worked as a domestic in a private house outside The Park in the 1950s. Afterwards attended the hospital industrial unit until her retirement at the age of seventy-five. Now attends on a voluntary basis, helping with tea breaks, washing up, etc. In 1984 she was transferred to a small flat in the hospital for rehabilitation. First attempt at living outside in flat with three others after sixty-one years of institutional life was not successful because of the incompatibility of the group. Transferred to a residential home in 1989.

Elsie Born 1920. Suffers from spinal curvature. Attended special school but was discharged just before she was sixteen years old as being incapable of receiving further benefit from special school. Able to read fairly well. Was admitted in 1936 following parents' separation and mother's deteriorating mental health. On mother's admission to hospital, application was made for her detention. Transferred from The Park to Abbey Grange in 1973. Joined her friend Doris in residential home in 1989.

Enid Born 1913. Lived at home with her parents who did not wish her to go to an institution. No attempt made to educate her at all, possibly because of her physical handicaps. She was unable to walk and had a curved spine. She was admitted in 1963 following the death of her mother because there was no-one to care for her. Attended the hospital training departments until her retirement in 1977. She had some difficulty speaking but made great efforts to be understood. She died in 1988 in The Park, peacefully in her sleep.

Ernest Born in 1928. Suffered from spina bifida. Was admitted to the local general hospital in 1938 because of neglect. Transferred from general hospital to The Park in 1945. No record of any education. Largely self-taught. Worked in the hospital departments and on the villa where his academic skills were useful in organising the clothing store. Described as 'the most intelligent patient in the hospital', he was asked to speak on behalf of other residents on formal occasions such as moving a vote of thanks to the Lord Mayor. He wrote his own account of life in The Park in 1974 which is in the hospital library. His physical health was poor and he became increasingly physically disabled, relying on a wheelchair during his last years. He was sustained by a deep religious faith and his close relationship with a fellow resident which lasted from 1971 until his death in August 1989.

Frank Born 1917. Attended a special school from age of eight to twelve years when he was discharged as ineducable. Afterwards attended a Junior Occupation Centre until 1932 when he was admitted following the death of his parents and the inability of his grandfather to care for him. He ran away a number of times. Developed arthritis in his late fifties and now has some difficulty in moving about. He became blind at the age of fifty-eight. He attended a centre for physically handicapped people outside the hospital for a few years before his retirement. He is very independently minded. He recently made his will and has expressed a strong desire to live outside The Park.

George Born 1942 with cerebral palsy. Unable to walk. Admitted in 1950 as being unable to be cared for at home. No record of any education outside or inside The Park. From the age of sixteen he worked in the industrial unit of the hospital and was valued as a quality checker. Highly motivated towards work and living outside and persistently requested both. Acquired an electric wheelchair in 1981. Speech difficult but he makes himself understood and became competent in symbolic language. Attempts to transfer him to a hostel for physically handicapped people failed. Eventually he was transferred to a workshop for physically handicapped people outside the hospital in 1984. He finally achieved his aim and now lives happily in a supported flat in the community with his friend Tom.

Grace Born 1915. Attended primary school to the age of ten years. Attended special school but was discharged at the age of fourteen and a half as being ineducable. Worked as a domestic but was unable to keep jobs. Attempted suicide at the age of sixteen (suicide was then an illegal act). Eventually admitted to The Park at the age of eighteen in 1933. While in The Park worked as a domestic in a local house for two and a half years. Ran away from The Park on at least one occasion. At the age of fifty-seven she was discharged into the community under the supervision of Social Services. She now lives alone in her own flat.

Henry Born 1924. He was illegitimate and deserted by his mother. He lived with foster parents who were paid 7s. 6d. per week for his keep. He went to special school at the age of six years but was discharged as ineducable after six months. He was admitted in July 1931 because he required greater supervision than his foster parents were able to provide. At the age of twenty he worked outside the hospital, labouring for a local baronet. Later worked on the villas. In 1974 identified as a potential hostel candidate. Transferred to the hospital training departments where he made progress in reading and writing. Transferred to a local authority hostel and training centre in 1975 after fifty-one years in The Park. His return visits to the hospital were discouraged. He still lives in the hostel with his friend Horace.

Horace Born 1922. Attended special school until the age of twelve, then went to Junior Occupation Centre for ineducable children. After this he worked in the tailoring department at an industry centre. He was admitted in 1939 at the age of seventeen. While in The Park he worked outside in a local clothing factory. He was transferred to a local authority hostel in 1970. Later moved to live in the same hostel as his friend Herbert in 1975. Still lives there.

Joan Born 1933. Has severe physical handicaps which affect muscle control throughout her body. Was admitted two weeks after her eighth birthday. She is very dependent on others for her physical needs. Very little is known of her early life. She was transferred to an adult villa in 1970. Has long-standing relationship with Margaret who helps her to communicate. Because of her physical problems, she's greatly troubled by chest infections. She makes considerable effort to be independent and co-operative and is very well liked in The Park. She has lived with a small group of close friends on a villa for many years.

Joe Born 1912. Attended special school for a few days when he was seven but was discharged as being incapable of benefiting from education at school. His parents was elderly and he was admitted in 1921 at the age of nine. There is no record of any education in The Park. He was greatly valued as a worker. He worked outside the hospital and a request was made by one of his friends outside in 1955 for him to work as a gardener. The institution did not consider this suitable. He had a paper round outside the hospital which he kept until 1979 when he gave it up because of his arthritis. He married a fellow resident in 1981 and was discharged into the community in 1982 to live in a flat with his wife. He died in a hospice in 1988.

Margaret Born in 1946. Has cerebral palsy and spent much of her early childhood in convalescent hospital. When her parents moved in 1951, she was admitted to The Park, at the age of five years. Attended the hospital therapy departments and was a Guide. Now works in the industrial unit and is a member of the Works Committee. Has her own electric wheelchair. Is a very good conversationalist and has a number of close friends. She is able to help Joan and one or two others communicate.

Sally Born 1924. Attended special school for six years until she was fourteen. At the age of seventeen, because she was unable to attend work regularly and frequently stayed out late, application was made for her detention. She was admitted in 1942. She was released on licence to live with an aunt 200 miles away in 1946. She helped to look after the children and grandchildren. She was returned to The Park in 1951, following an episode of depression. She made attempts to abscond and to injure herself. In 1969 she requested that the Mental Health Tribunal help her to find a job outside the hospital. She did have two domestic jobs which were short-lived. Attended a local authority training centre until her discharge in 1983, when she declined to attend further. She now lives on her own in a flat.

Tom Born 1936. No record of any education. Application for admission made by mother in 1946. In The Park, worked full-time in the ward kitchen for many years. Eventually moved to the industrial unit and from there to a Social Services training centre. Moved to a hospital flat in 1984 where he lived with his friend George until they moved together into a supported flat in the community in 1985.

Violet Born 1906. Attended a special school from the age of seven to sixteen years. Then occupied herself at home doing domestic tasks and knitting and sewing. Was admitted to The Park in 1934 following the death of her surviving parent. In The Park she did domestic work on the villa and sewing and helped considerably with other patients. She was still actively involved in these occupations when she was well over seventy. She died in The Park in 1988 of heart failure.

Index

Abbey Grange, 31, 51, 76
absconding, 62, 102
admission procedures, 13–14, 38
advocacy, 142
air raid, 101–2
assessment, 14, 15, 16, 19, 72, 137–8

barber, 55
bathtimes, 33, 54
bedtimes, 52
benefits trap, 139
birthdays, 97
Board of Control, 20, 23, 39, 69
bromide, 65, 67
bugle band, 91

certification, 18, 20, 21, 22, 35, 38
Chief Male Nurse, 32
children, 69, 85, 97, 136
Christmas, 93–7
church, 53, 90
cinema, 53, 86
clothing, 39, 40, 43, 52, 107
colony system, 26
community, 142
concerts, 53
conduct money, 60

dances, 89, 92
day-trips, 97–9
Dendy, Mary, 26
dental care, 55–6
discipline, 43; see also punishment
doctors, 57, 112–13
drugs, 65, 67, 68
dysentery, 34, 56, 57

education, 15, 69, 139
enemas, 57
epilepsy, 57
escape, 63, 64, 102
Executive Officer, 13, 14, 20–1

family, relationships with, 103–8

fancy dress dance, 87
farm, 51, 77, 78
feelings, 141
films, 53, 86–7
food, 44–5, 48–51
friendships, 109, 125

German prisoners of war, 33, 99–100
Girls Training Home, 25, 26
grounds, 35
Guides, 90–2
gymnastic displays, 91

haircuts, 40, 55
health care, 56, 57
Health Service Act 1948, 119
'high grades', 30, 136
holidays, 97–9
homosexuality, 117
hospital villa, 32, 57
human rights, 142

incontinence, 61
infections, 34, 56
infestations, 56
integration, 142

Junior Occupation Centres, 72

kindergarten, 69
kitchens, 74, 76, 78

laundry, 73, 74, 76
laxatives, 67
lesiure, 51, 83–99
local authorities, 20
'low grades', 30, 135

magistrates, 21
mail, censorship of, 42
market garden, 51, 78, 80
marriage, 116, 141
meals, 44–5, 48–51
medical care, 57

Medical Superintendent, 32, 57
medication, 57, 65, 140
Mental Deficiency Act 1913, 19, 20, 21, 22, 103
Mental Health Act 1959, 35, 119, 127, 139
money, 60, 62, 68, 77
moving out, 119–33

normalisation, 143
nurses, 111–12
nurses' home, 32, 74, 76

Oakwood, 27
offences, 60, 62
Orchards, The, 26, 27, 34, 51
overcrowding, 33, 34

paraldehyde, 67
parents, 103
parole, 22, 106–7
payment for work, 77, 79, 139
personal possessions, 38, 42
petition, 13
physically handicapped, 15, 16, 61, 81, 109
picture shows, 53, 86–7
presents, 95
Princess Royal, 32, 92
privacy, 41, 42, 119
privileges, 59, 60, 106, 140
punishment, 30, 43, 59–68, 140
punishment villa, 63, 64, 66

recreation hall, 32, 51, 53, 85–90
Recreation Hour, 83
relationships, 103–17, 141–2
religious services, 53, 89

school, 27, 32, 69, 70, 136
Scouts, 90–2
Second World War, 32, 33, 79, 99–102
sedatives, 67
self-sufficiency, 140
settling in, 40, 103

sewing room, 76
sexes, segregation of, 27, 32, 53, 89, 113–17, 141
sexual relationships, 30, 141
side-rooms, 30, 62, 63, 64, 65
soldiers, 33, 99–101
sport, 92–3
sports day, 93
staff, 67, 137; relationships with, 111–12
staff accommodation, 32
staff shortages, 34
Statutory Declaration, 13

tailoring, 79
teeth, 55–6
terminology, 35, 137
toys, 85

village community, 143
villa system, 27
violence, 66–7
visitors, 41, 53–4, 103–6
visits home, 106–8

war years, 79, 98, 99–102
weekends, 52
work, 40, 72–81, 139
'working girls', 39, 74, 76
workshops, 32

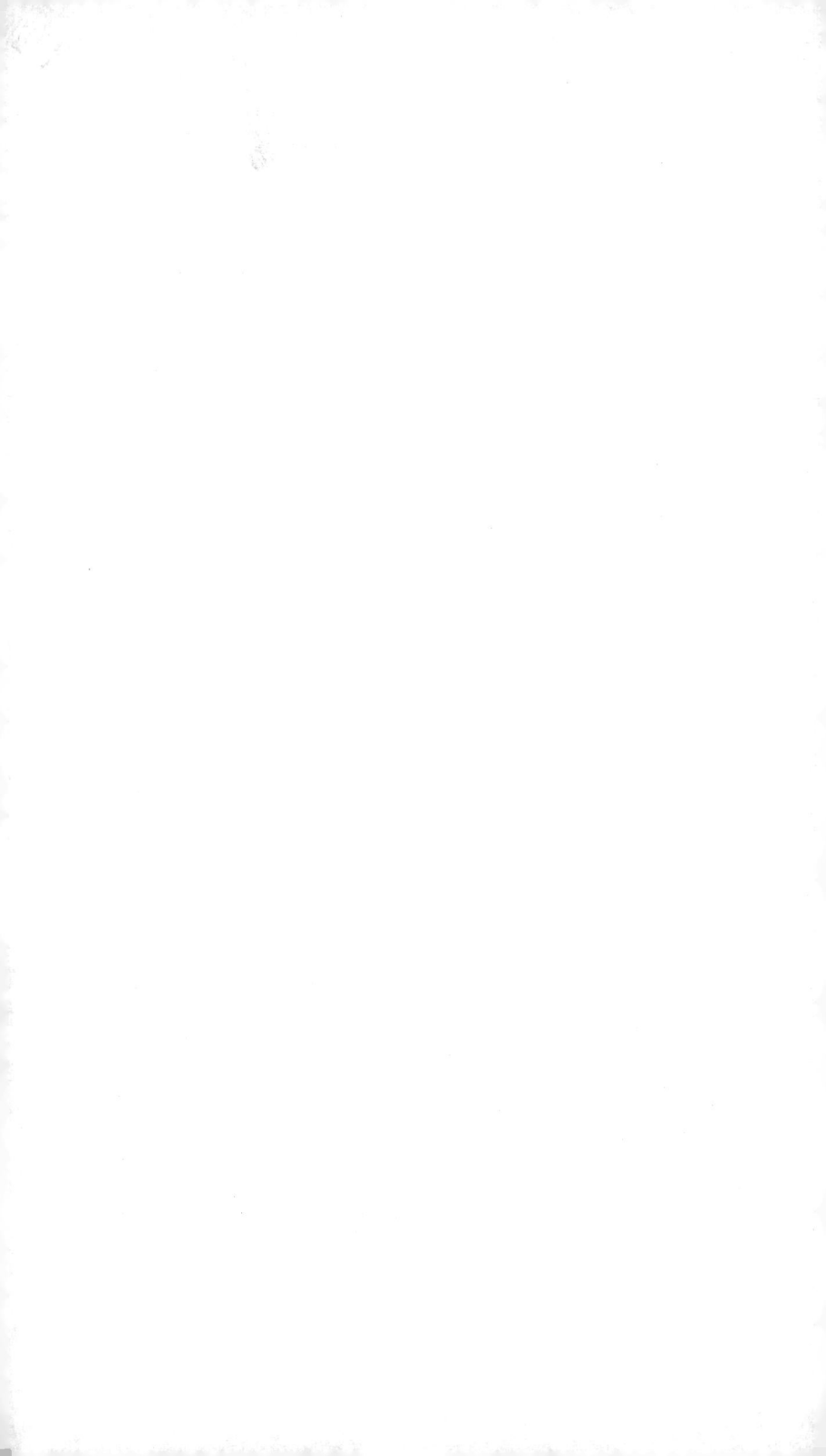

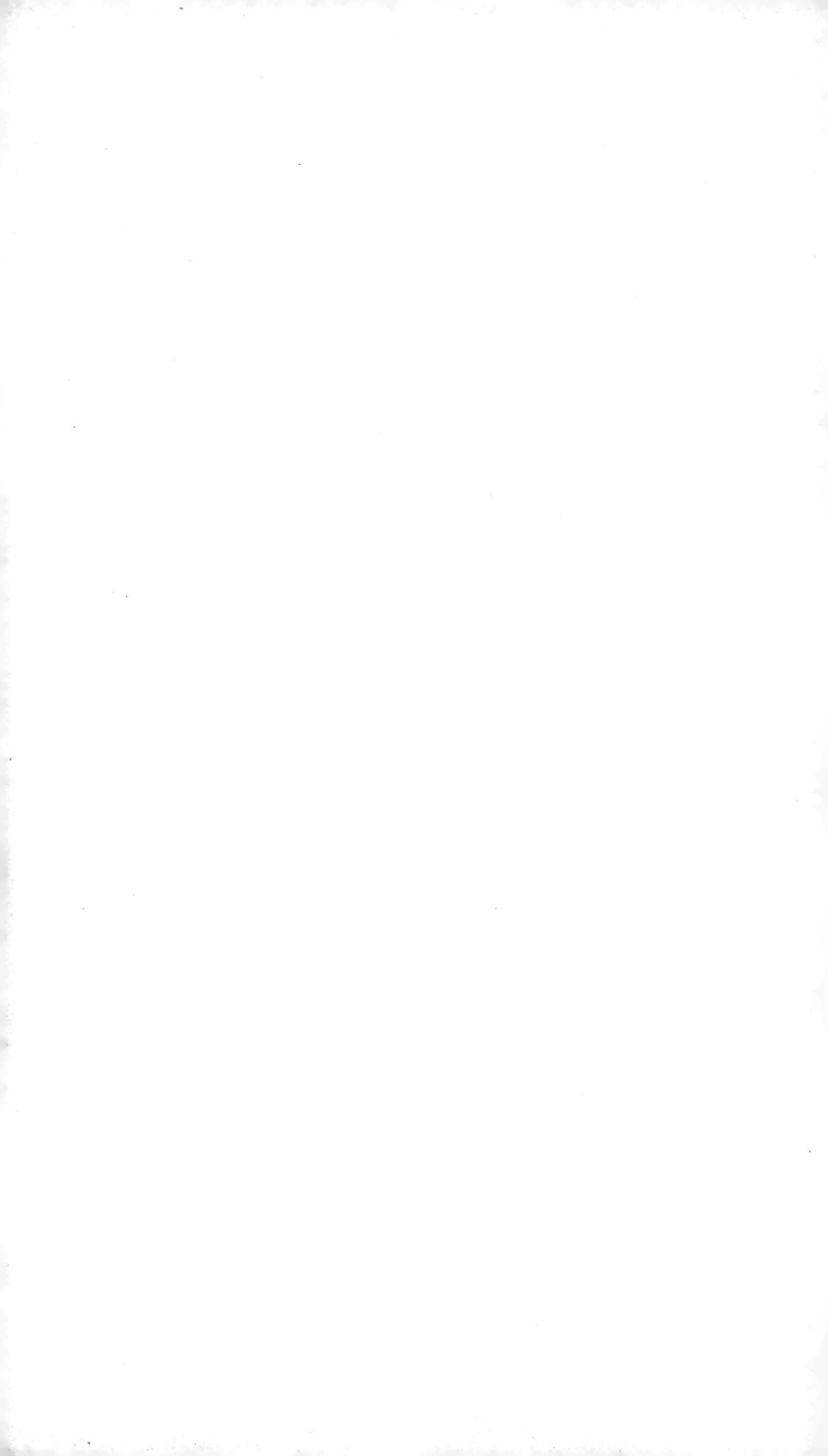